AN UNINTENDED JOURNEY

THE STORY OF ONE MAN'S
STRUGGLE WITH PROSTATE CANCER

Dick Grannan

Order this book online at www.trafford.com
or email orders@trafford.com

Most Trafford titles are also available at major online book retailers.

Printed in Victoria, BC, Canada.

ISBN: 978-1-4269-0387-8 (soft)
ISBN: 978-1-4269-0389-2 (ebook)

*Our mission is to efficiently provide the world's finest, most comprehensive book publishing
service, enabling every author to experience success. To find out how to publish your book, your
way, and have it available worldwide, visit us online at www.trafford.com*

Trafford rev. 12/01/2009

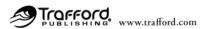 www.trafford.com

North America & international
toll-free: 1 888 232 4444 (USA & Canada)
phone: 250 383 6864 ♦ fax: 812 355 4082

*For the devoted medical
staff at Princess Margaret
Hospital, Toronto, Ontario*

Acknowledgements

Without the full-time support of my wife, Maureen, I would never have been able to complete this long and arduous journey. Her constant encouragement, bearing up under my 'don't give a shit' attitude, and her eternal love helped me stave off any descent into despair. Especially helpful was her attendance at the weekly medical meetings, where I was often too distraught to listen attentively, but she was there to provide the correct information I required later.

I would never have had the perseverance to complete this manuscript without the encouragement of my wife and many loyal friends. However, I owe special thanks to one editor at Nitpickers Proofreading and Editing in Toronto.

Thank You One and All

Introduction

You are about to share with me my incredible journey as I attempt to find my personal cure for prostate cancer.

Every family has been touched, in some way, by cancer. In the past such a horrible revelation was often secreted within the family circle, and discussed in hushed tones. It was considered a death notice, a matter of time. Conversations were often subdued, private and impregnated with the personal fear that someday they too might hear those awful words: '*You have cancer*'. Nobody wants to dwell on the cancer word, as if thinking about it might bring it on.

Thanks to modern medicine the senior population is becoming one of the largest units in our society, and that population is expected to double in the next three decades, from 4.2 million to 9.8 million. However, along with this growth comes the sad revelation for men that since 1987 there has been a 121.5% increase in prostate cancer cases. Literally thousands of unsuspecting men will hear those words in the next year, words they thought were surely meant for others, not for them. Shock and awe will be their immediate response.

Fortunately, now many prostate cancer patients who will take this passage return in good health. But there is still much to learn, and unfortunately, it still becomes a one-way trip for thousands of Canadians.

This book is an invitation to share my emotions, experiences, and even humorous situations, as I submit to months of treatments. This is not a medical book, but an intimate description of how it feels to put your future in the hands of others.

Dick Grannan

Diagnosed with prostate cancer in the spring of 2007 I had no idea that I was about to begin an incredible journey and meet so many amazing people, medical staff and friends, who would make every human effort to ensure a seat for me on the return trip.

Medical personnel were most helpful, explaining the disease and the different treatments I received. But no one was able to tell me why I was singled out, in the first place.

Most men, if they live long enough, will get clinically insignificant prostate cancer. However, about seventeen percent will end up with clinically significant prostate cancer like I did.

In her recent book *The Secret History of the War on Cancer,* Debra Davis says: "for hundreds of years we have known that smoking, hormones, bad nutrition, alcohol and bum luck, all affect the chance we will get cancer." In my case I guess it was just bum luck, or at least I might add old age to her list.

I found there was also an abundance of literature to help me understand this journey. Anyone who wishes to prepare himself for the experience and learn more, and has access to the Internet, will be surprised at the amount of safe information that can be found there. However, in spite of the plethora of material, there is a dearth of first person stories told by those of us who have been successfully treated. *An Unintended Journey* set out to remedy that lack.

It is one thing to learn the scientific facts about the various treatments available today and it is highly encouraged that you do so. However, to accompany me, a cancer patient, along the way will heighten and enrich your knowledge. By actually experiencing this journey with me, the medical explanations, test and treatment descriptions, and sometimes strange procedures will take on a new and more powerful meaning.

This was one journey I hoped I would never have to make. Many of my friends have traveled this busy way before me, some have returned to a richer and more meaningful life, but others were denied the joys of a return trip.

This is the story of my journey down the cancer thoroughfare and I hope it will assist you, as well as your partners, and your family, if you suddenly learn you too are about to make this unintended journey.

Dick Grannan

"If I knew I was going to live this long I would have taken better care of myself."

Groucho Marx

On October 30, 2006, my wife Maureen and I arrived at a parking lot near the Princess Margaret Hospital (PMH) in downtown Toronto. The warm afternoon sun made it feel like spring.

Driving in concentric circles in a nearby parking garage, we finally found a place to park on the sixth floor. Three cooing pigeons were perched on the cement rail, carefully preening themselves and ignoring the passing cars and pedestrians, as we walked to the nearby elevator. We took the scruffy and overworked conveyance to the street level.

As we emerged on the bottom floor, the Murray Street traffic resembled an Oriental bazaar, as cars, vans, delivery vehicles and construction equipment jockeyed for position, and pedestrians scurried in all directions.

The mild weather had melted an earlier snowfall and tiny rivulets trickled along the gutter making it necessary, in the midst of this confusion, to find a dry passageway on the west side of the street.

It was during my annual checkup on June 20, 2006, that my primary care doctor located some bumps on my prostate gland and decided that I should go for further testing. The earliest appointment he was able to make with a specialist at the Murray Koffler Urologic Wellness Centre in Toronto was in October, four months later.

The front door to the Koffler building opened into a steep set of stairs that led to the lobby and the bank of elevators. It was obviously an old building, but we could see workers on the outside completing what appeared to be a modern addition to the rear of the structure.

As we found our way to the office of the Erectile Dysfunction and Prostatitis Clinic on the sixth floor, we were astonished to see a major renovation had taken place. To our surprise, we entered a large and pleasant waiting room. We had expected the usual cramped sitting areas, with tables piled high with magazines two or three years old, and patients shuffling for seats.

This club-like space was bright and airy with comfortable leather chesterfields. Informative articles and brochures were neatly displayed on small tables or stands. Current health magazines were stacked on the coffee tables. The area was designed so that the patients were well spread throughout the room allowing maximum privacy while waiting for their appointment. A few couples were engaged in their own discussions or completing information sheets on clipboards. It was a vast improvement over the usual small, crowded waiting areas found in most medical offices.

The friendly official at the reception desk, after examining and recording my Health and Hospital Cards, handed me a questionnaire to be returned to her upon completion. My wife Maureen and I settled into one of the large coffee-colored leather couches, clipboard in hand, and I began ticking off the little boxes on the question sheet. The majority of the requests for information dealt with my dysfunctional urinary problems, such as the frequency of my nightly visits to the bathroom and the length of time it takes me to void my bladder. This apparently becomes a common problem for males over forty. They say one in four men will show these symptoms that are related to an enlarged prostate. I figured an average of two times a night was about right and checked the appropriate boxes. Although waking up each night was a nuisance, I was able to quietly sneak back to bed and was soon asleep. Maureen knew about my nightly crawls to the toilet, but I tried not to disturb her sleep when I slipped out of bed. There is a bathroom off our bedroom, but I usually walked down the hall to another one near the kitchen, so that the trickle of running water, slowly dribbling into the bowl, would not spoil her sleep. I simply attributed my nightly ambles to the aging process and did not give it another thought until confronted by the clipboard questions in the doctor's plush waiting area. As we sat comfortably on the large sofa, smiling as we discussed the appropriate answer to each query, I suddenly realized they must have a serious purpose, otherwise why was this information important?

That was the easy part as the second page of questions became very personal. I suddenly felt uneasy having Maureen helping me with the answers. It is one thing to talk about my middle-of-the-night trips to pee, but the second page was soliciting information about my sperm. Slightly embarrassed, and with less consultation with Maureen, I quickly ticked off the boxes. My theory was that at my age, seventy-eight-years old, the best I could say was the supply seemed to be getting pretty low. The delivery system was still intact, but the source in the warehouse was definitely waning. How I knew that information will remain a mystery, and Maureen was discreet enough not to ask.

After answering truthfully, I returned the completed questionnaire to the assistant at the front desk and retreated to our spot on the chesterfield. I kept peeking over to see if she was reading my answers to page two of the questionnaire. A half hour later a doctor appeared in a large open doorway a good distance from where we were sitting. I guessed him to be in his late forties, tall and wearing the prescribed doctor's white lab coat. He had a full head of black hair and wore glasses. In his left hand he clutched the clipboard containing my answer sheets. Glancing down he read my name off his clipboard, and then looked up to see who would respond. I identified myself with a wave of my hand. Maureen and I stood up gathering our belongings into our arms. He asked us to follow him around the corner and down the hall. We entered a small, but sterile office. It appeared not to be a private office, but a common office used for interviews. I placed my leather jacket over the back of my chair while Maureen kept hers on her lap. We sat down facing the doctor who was already busy shuffling through the questionnaire making short notations here and there. We were anxious to find out why my GP had sent me here. Experiencing a little trouble with my bladder and apparently developing a few bumps on my prostate was no big deal. However, I noticed, as I placed my jacket behind me on the chair, that he gave me a strange look, which I interpreted to mean *don't settle in*. I took the look as a hint that we needed to move quickly and that his time was extremely important. The doctor was apparently all business. I thought of something I recently read about the Ontario's *Six Principles of Health*, the number one principle being: "Keep Patient Front and Centre." Rightly or wrongly I jumped to the conclusion that time and workload, not front and center, were the driving forces here.

He was there, not to engage in idle chat with Maureen and me, but to gather medical facts. Turning his office into an assembly line may be a practical approach, but it was one sure way to destroy communication and I immediately felt unwelcome and unsatisfied. I was not off to a very good start.

He asked a few preliminary questions assuring himself I was the same individual whose name was inscribed on his clipboard. He did not follow the usual procedure, or refer to a file folder of previous records, as far as I could determine. He then asked me to follow him, alone, to a small examination room down the hall and around another corner. I was asked to lower my pants and underwear and lie on my left side, knees up to my chin, on the paper covered examination table. He then immediately administered the first of many similar examinations, the somewhat embarrassing and dreaded Digital Rectal Examination (DRE). It's probably not the high point in the urologist's day either. He then informed me that my prostate was indeed enlarged and that he had detected a number of bumps.

The prostate is made up of two zones: the outer layer or peripheral, and the central or transitional inner layer. As men get older the transition zone gets larger until it becomes the largest zone of the prostate and it is there that cancer is likely to get its start in life. Since this zone is next to the rectum, the doctor can put on his rubber gloves and search around with his finger. The prostate is usually smooth, so if anything feels different, such as bumps, it becomes a starting point. Obviously this preliminary examination of the prostate is the doctor's *à notre façon*, the way they do it and probably has an element of subjectivity. As I cannot watch this procedure, for obvious reasons, I am not sure exactly which digit is involved, but I suspect it is the one commonly used to salute an offending driver. Not to worry, the hand was gloved and the glove was well lubricated. TV personality Howie Mandel, when asked about a trip to the proctologist, asked how could you know for certain if your prostate is enlarged? "Maybe," he said, "the doctor just had a long finger."

Upon completion of this uncomfortable, and somewhat obscene prod, we went back to the first office, where Maureen was quietly waiting. Without saying a word he penned instructions for a number of procedures. We then followed him, like grade school kids, to the front desk where he gave his notes to the secretary and left.

He ordered the usual blood and urine tests, and his assistant arranged dates for a Cystoscopy and an abdominal and prostate Ultrasound. He also prescribed Flomax CR controlled-release tablets to deal with the symptoms I had described on the clipboard. The drug is used primarily for Benign Prostatic Hyperplasia (BPH) to help control the flow of urine and nourish the sperm. The early assumptions being that the growth bumps are benign, that they are neither cancerous nor will they lead to cancer, but are obstructing the bladder. I love the warnings that accompanied the leaflets provided by the pharmacist when I picked up my first box of Flomax at the pharmacy.

"Extremely rarely, FLOMAX Capsules and similar medications have caused prolonged, painful erection of the penis, which is unrelieved by sexual intercourse or masturbation. This condition, if untreated, can lead to permanent inability to have an erection. If you suspect such symptoms, call your doctor or go to an Emergency Room as soon as possible."

I am still trying to figure out exactly how I would approach the triage nurse, and what I would whisper in her ear, when I reached the hospital emergency room if confronted with this side effect.

2

We left his office a little bewildered and I still felt we were not communicating. The doctor was all business and definitely not loquacious. This was a new experience for me. I usually leave a doctor's office with some sense that the problem has been identified and a course of action has been prescribed. Sometimes common sense and reason is blurred by belief or custom. We were brought up to believe that if you had a health problem you went to the doctor's office, and if necessary to the hospital, to have it fixed. Like taking a car or a broken radio to the shop for repairs. Experience has often proved differently, but the old beliefs and expectations seem to linger on. I later realized of course, the problem has to be identified and this visit was the first step in the search for answers. Since the problem was not clear, more research was necessary and he was bent on finding out what was going on.

Nonetheless, I did not think of this experience as being a visit to the doctor's office in the traditional sense as it felt more like a quick shuffle around two tiny examination rooms. Before we left the front desk, where the secretary was processing the appointments for my tests, the doctor was again standing at the open doorway, his clipboard in hand, his white coat in place, reading the next name from his clipboard and peering around at the waiting patients, hoping to identify his next appointment. I was just another client in his long and busy day.

This was the beginning of the long wait. The blood and urine donations were completed that same day in the lab two floors down. However, the next test, the Cystoscopy, a visual examination of the bladder and its outlet, in my case read penis, was scheduled for

November 27, 2006. The abdominal Ultrasound was arranged for December 4, 2006.

All this sudden action got me wondering. The first thing I decided to do was to learn something about the tests he had prescribed. The blood test included a PSA or Prostate-Specific Antigen reading. This antigen is not the same as the Microsoft antivirus and anti spam manager, but a small protein molecule produced by the prostate and is normally at a very low level in the blood stream where it can be measured. Anything under 4 ng/mL (nanograms per millilitre) is usually considered normal and anything over 10 ng/mL is high. After the magic age of forty-five most men should have this blood test performed. Recent statistics, however, show that only 39% of Canadian men bother to have this test according to an article in the *Globe and Mail*. Granted, this blood test is not perfect, but it's a start. One of the little vials they filled during my annual checkup visits to my GP was for that purpose, I presume. However, I was never given a specific number nor was it clear to me that the PSA reading had anything to do with cancer. Perhaps ignorance is truly bliss. Unfortunately, many men will develop cancer of the prostate if they live long enough. In many cases it will not be clinically significant, but for about 17% of us it will be. They say it takes eight to ten years for the cancer to become life threatening if not treated. So the lucky ones will die of something else during what is called the watchful waiting period.

The function of the prostate, deep in the pelvic area, is to make part of the seminal fluid that mixes with the sperm, to make semen, the stuff of ejaculations. This sugar-based substance provides energy to the sperm so they can chase after the female eggs. At the same time small amounts are released into the blood stream. However, when there is a problem with the prostate, more and more amounts are discharged into the blood leading to a higher PSA score. As well, some prostate cancer cells produce more enzymes than normal cells. Eventually, the protein can be detected in the blood stream. It is a clue that something may be wrong, remembering, of course, there is no magic number. Since PSA gradually rises with age the reading is often also age-adjusted. However, there can be other causes such as obesity, inflammation, infection and even sex. For a man in his 40s the cut off would be around 2.5 ng/mL.

For someone my age about 6.5 ng/mL would be an expected reading. Knowing that means they are less likely to get a false reading.

Suddenly, my research on the subject introduced me to the possibility that they were looking for cancer. The thought was probably in the back of my mind, but the brain refused to let it surface to the level of consciousness. Up until now, no one had even mentioned that miserable word to me. At the same time it was beginning to dawn on me that doctors are human; they don't have all the answers right away, and can't always fix whatever is broken. Besides they were not going to pop the cancer word before they had some certainty. So suddenly I was beginning to ask myself: was my prostate just getting old like its owner or, was there something more seriously scary going on? Obviously the doctor was not going to raise the cancer scare unless he had sufficient evidence to do so. And so began my unintended journey.

3

What I learned from this doctor was that he needed to gather as much information as he could and then, and only then, would he have something to discuss. What I learned from my reading, prior to the prescribed tests, was the possibility that Mr. C might be choosing another victim, namely me. Wisely, the doctor knew that if he mentioned the cancer word too early, he would only be raising unnecessary anxiety on our part. So I went ahead on my own and introduced my mind to the notion that this dreadful disease might have my name attached to it. Was I going to die soon? So much for avoiding unnecessary anxiety, I did that to myself without his help.

Most of us don't think much about our own death. Suddenly, it's back on my mind. As an article in *Maclean's* magazine pointed out: "Death goes against the spirit of the age." And Woody Allen once remarked: It's not that he was afraid to die, he just didn't want to be there when it happened. Although we all get a good dose of death through our daily news fix, those deaths are always about other unfortunate people. There seems to be a war raging somewhere, a plane crash, a collapsing bridge or high-rise, earthquakes and tsunamis, daily stabbings and shootings, and of course the numerous traffic accidents on our overcrowded and stressed-out highways. Because we see so much of it, the pictures become commonplace, part of our daily experience in this high tech world. Hence, they lack any deep impact. The exposure to this violence rarely promotes thoughts about our own inevitable demise, however. We are just too busy living our own lives and trying to survive one day at a time. After all, thanks to modern medicine,

I have already lived longer than my father who died at seventy-five. In the 1700's the average death for men was around forty. So we are almost doubling that average.

Like many people I had experienced some teachable moments about the finality of death. As a small boy growing up in the Maritimes, I first confronted death when my paternal grandmother died. As was the custom, she was waked for three days in our front living room. The only impact on me, however, was to avoid that part of the house, especially after dark.

My second experience with death was more personal. During early adolescence some well-meaning clergyman gathered the grade seven and eight boys together and informed us that masturbation was a mortal sin. We were told, that if we masturbated we would be condemned to hell for all of eternity. I was not even sure I knew what he was talking about at the time, but I sure did not want to die and go to hell forever.

Not long after that afternoon session in the local church hall, I was returning from a swim in the Fisher Lakes in Rockwood Park, where I learned from my grade six intelligentsia buddies, what the clergyman was talking about. Their profound words for this male practice were: *jerking off*.

We were returning through the bush and suddenly, sitting off the trail and probably believing he had complete privacy, was a young boy energetically pulling his pud. I wondered what he was doing? When I asked my chums there was a great deal of snickering as they explained to me, in great detail, what the young lad was about. Needless to say the boy engaged in self-abuse interrupted his pleasure and stomped off through the bush pulling up his pants. I thought the poor kid was probably going to die soon and go straight to hell. Not knowing what my peers knew, left me embarrassed and feeling estranged. The same feelings I was now having about my lack of knowledge of prostate cancer.

In late adolescence my third experience with death emerged from the horrors of the Second World War. I began to wonder why there was so much bad stuff going on in the world. "Mom," I remember asking, "aren't the German people just like our family, I don't understand?" I tried to be rational most of the time, but there had to be a way for people to get along with each other, all the killing and pain did not make sense to me. Although I did not realize it at the time, I was probably asking myself the great-unanswered question: what does it mean to be human? Better still, what is the purpose of my life? Alan Alda, of M*A*S*H* fame, once said in a radio interview in Toronto, that tackling the 'What's the meaning of my life' question in college was quixotic. A few years after the horrors of the Second World War some of us, as young as we were, did not think such thoughts were either rash or romantic. What in the hell were we doing to each other? Too many young men, some of them relatives, never came home. I remember sitting behind our house, during the war years, and thinking about the young men who had gone overseas and did not return. I knew families on our street, Rockland Road in Saint John, New Brunswick, who had lost a father, or a brother in Europe. Walking home in the early evening, after a game of ice hockey on Lily Lake, I would see the light in the window of a home where I knew a terrible loss had been experienced. Another familiar face would never join us again in a pick-up game of shinny on the lake. Many of them were just a few years older than me. Even though we lived in Canada, World War II touched us more deeply than the television wars of today. We felt more deeply the horrors of mass destruction of cities and the loss of so many friends and family because many were from our very neighborhood.

A more recent life-altering event was a sailing trip across the Atlantic Ocean in 1996. Some evenings, I would point to the stars, and say to a fellow crew member: "Did you ever stop to think that we may be nothing but ticks on the back of some cosmic cow?" I soon learned that this was a discussion he would rather avoid, especially when thirty-foot waves were bouncing us around. Spending weeks on a small sailboat, in the middle of the vast and often stormy ocean, drives home the most fundamental truth of all. It sits at the root of everyday existence. Everything we do, I learned far out on the stormy Atlantic, even when we are not aware of it, is for one purpose and one purpose only: to live and to survive as long as we can.

In the late fall of 2006 Laura Gainey, daughter of the General Manager of the Montreal Canadiens, was washed overboard from the three masted barque Picton Castle. At the time of this writing the event was still being investigated. However, I can relate to the incident as something similar happened to me. On that same trip across the ocean, late one evening, I was in the galley cleaning up after dinner. Suddenly, there was a banging on the hatch and Peter, the single crew member on deck-watch at the time, asked for help recovering the jib, or foresail, which had become loose. He had to go forward to the very front of the boat, retrieve the lines that held the jib sail, and lead them back to the cockpit. A very dangerous procedure on a small boat in the middle of the North Atlantic.

Our rule was never go on deck without being tethered to the boat. However, since my services were only required for a minute or two, I climbed up into the cockpit without my harness and leaned on the safety lines on the starboard side ready to receive the jib line Peter had retrieved from the bow of the boat. I had to then run it through the block on the deck where I was sitting, wrap it around a winch and secure it to a cleat. After that, I could return to the cabin.

As I completed the task, Peter went forward again to lead the loose port line back along that other side of the boat. Just as I finished cleating the line an extra large wave struck the vessel. I was lifted off the deck by the rushing water and thrown half way through the lifelines. My whole upper body was hanging over the side and I was being dragged overboard by the oncoming waves rushing past the boat. Fortunately, at the very last moment I managed to grab the lower lifeline with my left hand and was able to drag myself through it and back into the cockpit. It was a dark night, the waves were well over ten feet, and the surface was streaked with white caps. If I had fallen completely into the water neither Peter, nor the Skipper, who was asleep below, would have known. I would have been lost forever in the night. There are times when breaking the rules can result in disaster. I was plain lucky. That experience taught me never to stick my head out of the hatch without my tether, but more significantly, I learned how important survival is and how life can be stolen away in an instant.

Suddenly, my research on cancer presented the possibility of my own imminent death. Was I being dragged into a raging sea without a lifeline? The chance that I might have cancer, threatened to take away my freedom to be and my efforts to survive would become useless. Was some other force, bad luck or series of coincidences, taking over the writing of my life story? Was I entering the final stage? Was the Grim Reaper sharpening his scythe and searching me out?

Perhaps I should not have allowed the word cancer to strain my imagination until there was proof those ugly cells had colonized. I read that a man can have an enlarged prostate (BPH), with no evidence of a cancer. The prostate becomes larger and can obstruct the bladder. If the symptoms, for example, frequent waking up at night to pee, or the inability to urinate, interfere with life, there are treatments available. Besides the usual assortment of drugs to deal with this problem, there are methods that simply shrink the size of the enlarged prostate using a laser or using modern microwave technology. At one time they used a telescopic knife inserted through the urethra to core out the prostate. Thank God for advances in health care. I hoped my problem would turn out to be BPH and I need not have been so worried about the possibility of cancer.

I began to realize that there is a lot of scientific uncertainty about cancer, and I needed a lot more information before I panicked. I hoped that the prescribed tests would produce some useful data for the doctor. Once the information was in his possession I presumed something substantial would result for us to talk about. Meantime, the element of terror had been aroused by my research. I knew there was a real possibility that something might be seriously wrong with me.

4

On November 27, 2006, we arrived at Mount Sinai to see a specialist for the Cystoscopy. To say I enjoyed the Cystoscopy would be an exaggeration and may brand me as some sort of pervert. However, it was not what I expected.

We arrived at the waiting room ahead of the scheduled appointment, hoping things would move quickly. You would think by this time, and at my age and experience, I would know that things do not move promptly in hospitals, unless there is an emergency. There was something else I needed to learn at that time. After twelve years of retirement I was pretty much in control of my time. No rushing to the office in the mornings for a nine o'clock appointment; no supervisor looking over my shoulder. These frequent visits to the hospital were invading my precious freedom and I was convinced it would prove to be a difficult transition to conform to any new routine that might evolve.

We checked in on the first floor and provided the required identity and information for the computer records. Then we were directed to an upper floor waiting room. This section of Mount Sinai Hospital was so crowded it resembled a boarding lounge in a modern airport. One lady sitting next to us was quilting. Others were knitting. Still other patients were reading books, or anxiously paging through the tattered and outdated magazines. Backpacks and small bags were pushed under the seats. Obviously, many had learned from previous experience and came prepared for the inevitable. It was a mixture of patients hoping to get in for a procedure, but at the same time prepared to wait, accompanied by their friends or loved ones who had come to offer support. At one point an elderly man complained in a loud voice, and inquired why a late arrival was selected before him. The harassed young lady who was calling the patients into the treatment room was doing her best to mollify his outburst and explain to him the nature of emergencies.

We quickly realized it was going to take a long time and wished we had brought along our own reading material. For three hours we watched the restless patients shuffle back and forth to the washroom or we eavesdropped on the brief consultations being held in the hall nearby.

This experience also taught us that the time assigned on the posted printed appointment sheet, and which we had to confirm on the first floor entrance area, had little meaning on this floor. Patients were called on the basis of their reporting to the desk in this area and, not necessarily according to the time slotted on their appointment sheet down stairs. The moral of that story was come early.

A few years ago, when traveling in Rome with a tour group, we were attempting to cross the street near Vatican City. Cars were rushing back and forth oblivious to the changing traffic lights. When we questioned our tour guide as to why they were not stopping at the red light and letting us cross, he replied in his beautiful melodious Italian accent: *"Red lights are only a suggestion."* We felt the appointment time we were given down stairs must also have been only a suggestion.

Finally, my turn came and I was ushered into a small change room and asked to remove everything and don a hospital gown making sure it opened in the front. The assistant then secured my clothes in a locker. There were two other patients in this tiny inner room, another man and a young woman. Not knowing what to expect, and all three of us now clad in very loose, short, striped, standard hospital gowns, generated some attempts at humor, no doubt, to assuage the tension in the very small room. Anticipation of over exposure in a new and strange environment was obviously on everyone's mind.

When my name was called we moved into the procedure area. The assistant nurse helped me climb up on the angled table enabling me to observe her prep work. Without any hesitation she threw open my gown and, taking my penis in hand, she applied an anodyne, or local anesthetic, to the opening of the urethra, the narrow tube that runs the length of the penis. She used a needle to numb the area for a few minutes while the tube is eased into place.

As mentioned, a Cystoscopy is a procedure that makes it possible for the urologist to see into the urethra, prostate and urinary bladder. To do this a thin, flexible tube, called a cystoscope is inserted through the urethra and into the bladder to check for any abnormalities. If any trouble is spotted the doctor can actually remove small pieces of tissue for analysis and even crush small bladder stones if present. When I was properly prepared, the doctor, followed by six medical students, approached the bottom end of the table. Some time earlier I had been informed that this was a teaching hospital, but this was the first time I ended up center stage with my naked legs spread-eagle. I was happy to see they were all men.

However, my attention was quickly drawn away from the spectators and my eyes were drawn to a colored monitor that the doctor had angled halfway up the procedure table. In this position everyone present, including me, could observe the procedure on the monitor. My loss of modesty was forgotten as the doctor inserted the cystoscope and began his commentary for the students.

How often does anyone get the chance to take a trip through the inside of his own penis. We traveled up this beautiful pink tunnel until we came to a blockage. The urologist said we were approaching the muscle (urinary sphincters) that controls the bladder. It was closed and he had to push his way past. We then entered the bladder. It was mostly empty as we began the tour around the inside. Then sterile warm water was passed through the tube expanding the bladder, and we explored this new and fascinating world together.

Unfortunately, no one clapped at the end of my first TV performance. When I was asked to step down from the table a large towel was provided to collect the copious amounts of water that came with the extracted magic wand. Clinging to the towel I had to maneuver my way through the clutch of viewers as they whispered their observations to each other. As I was leaving the area they began moving into the show next door.

To this day I have no idea what this test, if anything, revealed. My untrained eye did not observe any problems, nor did the commentary reveal anything serious. I presumed nothing of interest was discovered and put the experience down as my taking part in an exciting voyage inside my own body.

Eight days later on December 4, 2006, I was ready for the next exciting adventure, the prostate Ultrasound. I must admit this one caught me off guard. After the colorful trip provided by the Cystoscopy, I was expecting something similar.

Often TV medical dramas will include an ultrasound segment. For example, an ER episode peeks in on an expectant mother-to-be. The viewer can see the tiny fetus pulsating in the black, white and grey environment. Having observed ultrasound sessions on the tube I was led to believe that it would be a painless experience. The technician would be using high-frequency sound waves to produce pictures in black, white and grey, much like sonar used by fishermen. Along with the electronics there is a scanner and a transducer, a small hand-held device attached to a cord. Ultrasound gel would be applied to my skin to help transmit the sound waves from the transducer to my internal organs. The device is moved around projecting pictures on the screen.

Once again I was given a gown and then ushered into a darkened room. Most of the gowns provided so far could be classified as reasonable. On at least one occasion I was offered one that was far too small and I had difficulty protecting my privacy. However, some places provide gowns with names like Tropical Breeze, Blue Lagoon or Pink Flowers. What would I have done if I were handed the Pink Flowers version? I presume they save those for their female customers. The most I have seen were a light blue, or grey, with vertical prison stripes.

I was asked to get on a table next to the ultrasound equipment, and to lie on my back. My short gown was thrown open and the technician smeared some gel over my lower stomach and pelvis girdle and began moving the transducer. In the beginning it was indeed painless just as I had seen it on TV. Unfortunately, I was unable to see the video screen as it was mounted high on my right side. He was seated in such a way as to block my vision and at the same time watch both the screen and my body. This was a disappointment after the Cystoscopy show. When I did get a chance to peek, it was mostly colorless images I could not identify. The technician was not the garrulous type and no commentary was forthcoming. I decided to let him do his job and not ask questions he was not interested in answering.

He spent about twenty minutes going over and over the same locations. When he stopped he said he would be leaving the room for a few minutes. He asked me to roll over and lay on my left side with my knees slightly drawn up facing the wall, a position I was becoming accustomed to. It prompted me to ponder that since patients spend a lot of time on their back facing the acoustic ceilings tiles, or blank walls, perhaps some pictures, would help dispel some of the anxiety by distracting the mind.

Just before he left the room however, and while I was facing the wall, I hear a sound of rubber being pulled over an object. After he left, and I was sure he was not close by, I rolled back to try to see what he had done. There attached to the ultrasound machine was another kind of transducer, a rod about the size of a middle finger, and he had pulled a condom over it. The transducer probe pointing ominously at the ceiling looked as if someone was giving me the finger. Suddenly, my heart began to thump. I had a good idea where he was going to poke that rod when he came back.

When I heard him returning to the semi-dark room, I dutifully rolled back on my left side and assumed my position facing the wall. He sat down and immediately eased the finger-like transducer into place and began moving it around in my rectum. The reflected sound waves would show the size of the enlarged prostate and if there was any abnormal growth that might indicate cancer was present. After the Cystoscopy, this was indeed a bummer. It was not a pleasant experience and I was happy when he finished and told me to get dressed. I could not don my clothes fast enough and Maureen and I left the building posthaste to get something to eat. I was definitely looking for a place where I could stand up. I presume the urologist got the results, but no one ever reported them to me.

5

By early December I figured they must have enough information to let me in on the consequences. The results were available from the DRE, the PSA, the Cystocopsy and the Ultrasound. My next appointment with the doctor was December 14, 2006. Once again we found a parking space near the Murray Koffler Family Centre and proceeded to the now familiar waiting area on the sixth floor.

Still clinging to his clipboard and, dressed in his traditional white lab coat, the urologist appeared at the open doorway and summoned us to the same little office. I kept my coat over my arm this time. He had a small folder on the desk in front of him, containing, I presume, the results of the tests he had ordered. I was anxious to hear the conclusions. He silently made a few notes and checked off a number of items. I supposed this was the first opportunity he had to examine the reports. Then, without any preliminaries, or revealing any test results, he looked up and verbally delivered some upsetting news: He told me that I had a 50/50 chance that cancer is present in my prostate. Wham!!!

The physical response to a life-threatening event is referred to as the 'fight or flight syndrome'. It is a primitive reaction when the danger is perceived as a certain defeat. Unfortunately, the word cancer, no matter which variety, has an element of defeatism inherent in it. In fact, the old *Webster's Seventh New Collegiate Dictionary* includes the definition: 'a source of evil'.

Some people describe such occasions of shock, as having a sinking feeling. A wave of some sort passed through my whole being as my heartbeat significantly increased. I suddenly found it hard to breathe and my mouth became very dry. All of my blood vessels must have closed up at once and my skin tingled as if I was struck by lightning. I could feel the hair rising on the back of my neck. For a moment I was stunned. My body was marshalling its primal defenses and at the same time I was attempting to hide from the doctor and my wife, what was happening to me.

At this early juncture in my journey the little information I had gathered was purely cerebral. I had not internalized it emotionally. Although it was a worry on my mind, I had not allowed it to sink below my neck nor did I totally embrace the full impact of the 'C' word. It was all a mental exercise. Suddenly, one sentence from this doctor and the information is no longer just theory. He was talking about me and not someone else. I quickly tried to console myself with the thought that he said there was a 50% chance I had cancer, meaning there was also a 50% chance that I did not.

All year long we are asked to support hundreds of different events to help raise funds for a cancer cure. There are runs, lotteries, donations at wakes, and ads on TV all saying one thing: "We do not have a cure for cancer." Suddenly, everything changes. This disease, for which they have not yet found a cure, according to the ads and promotions, now has a hold on me. I have heard that it can be put off with treatment until I die of some other cause. My hope was that the cancer could be reasonably controlled through treatment for as long as possible. I was certain that I did not wish to be subject to futile treatments, if it should come to that. Thus, the magnitude and depth of my reaction. The doctor seemed unaware of the jolt I had experienced, or if he was aware, he ignored the signs and went on with his recommendations.

Dr. Groopman M.D., of Harvard Medical School points out in his book *How Doctors Think*: "Recently there have been great clinical successes against types of cancers that were previously intractable, but many malignancies remain that can be, at best, only temporarily controlled. How an oncologist thinks through the value of complex and harsh treatments demands not only an understanding of science but also a sensibility about the soul, how much risk we are willing to take and how we want to live out our lives."

An enlarged prostate, I had already learned, causes a number of socially embarrassing situations, none of which is life threatening. Two major social difficulties had become apparent to me in the past year.

First, what I call the loss of Directional Control. Imagine this: at intermission in a theater you walk into the men's room and take your place, shoulder to shoulder, with the row of gentlemen already facing the wall. For some reason it is becoming more and more difficult to start the flow, especially in a public place. I have observed that if there is no reading material, such as the daily Sports Page or TV screen attached to the wall, men modestly focused down to observe the accuracy of the flow and to protect their shoes. Rarely do they look sideways or engage in conversation with the man at the next urinal. To engage in conversation, while standing in a public place holding on to your exposed penis, could easily be misinterpreted. Finally, after much effort, you get the flow working when you suddenly discover, to your horror, that you are producing, not one, but two lines of fire, endangering each of your neighbors. The Tigris River is off to the right, and the Euphrates River off to the left. Since men are not equipped with dual-control you must first stop the stream and wait a few seconds to start again. When you are finally able to sneak a look, left and right along the line, you discover all new faces. The boys in the waiting line must be wondering why I am taking so long.

The second major difficulty is the Oops Factor: This is especially annoying in the summer time when you are wearing light colored pants and even worse if you are wearing shorts. When your task is complete, or so you believe, you zip-up and head for the sink to wash your hands. Suddenly, there appears a large spot in the crotch of your pants. Post-voidal drip has caught you unawares. Your salvation rests with the hot air hand drier, if you are lucky enough to find one. Otherwise, you have to do a lot of daubing and fanning with a paper towel. I finally decided the best course of action in these public situations, was to just wait longer at the urinal.

I had no idea that my prostate was growing and putting the squeeze on my urethra causing this loss of control. I just thought it was another nugget sent to enhance my Golden Years. I considered these difficulties merely one more problem to make my life more exciting. That there might be cancer hiding there, prior to my beginning this journey, never entered my mind.

At the end of this second visit with the doctor we again went to the front desk to discover he had ordered a second ultrasound but this time to include a biopsy. This biopsy is known as a TRUS or Transrectal Ultrasound (with Biopsy). Since the DRE and PSA alone cannot signal cancer, they can indicate that there is a need for a biopsy. At least by then I knew what to expect with yet another expedition into that nether region of my body that does not see a lot of sunlight. God, getting a cast on a broken wrist is so much easier.

6

On January 24, 2007, we went once again to the hospital for the second Transrectal Ultrasound of the Prostate (TRUS), but this time to include a biopsy. The procedure is done to see if samples of the prostate gland are cancerous and to learn why the PSA was high. I was sent to a special waiting room marked *Men Only* while Maureen found her way to the general sitting area. After I was properly gowned, I entered the small room and joined two other men anticipating the same procedure. A young woman came into the room and called my name. I followed her into a small office. She sat me down and asked a number of similar questions to the ones I had first encountered in the previous lobby-like antechamber at the Koffler Centre. Considering the age of the young woman, I had to be brave when she got to the questions about the ancillary functions the male organ is capable of performing.

I returned to the antechamber where a small television played in the corner and a few outdated magazines were available on a coffee table. An elderly gentleman, and a student from the University of Toronto, both volunteers, were near the change rooms looking after our needs and protecting our clothes. (I was told to leave my wallet with Maureen.) I was reading a magazine article when a patient exited the procedure rooms, looked at us, as he clasped his robes about him, and said: "I hope I never have to do that again." That was a real morale buster.

Finally, my name was called and I was told to make one last trip to the bathroom, where I was unable to produce any results. I returned to the treatment room and the doctor came to prepare his equipment and to get me to sign the consent form. He asked if I had taken antibiotics for the past three days as prescribed. Again I had to assume a senior fetal position on my left side. By now they really did not have to tell me what to do. It was my privilege to stare at the cream-colored wall again waiting for my butt to become the area of critical attention.

He then cleaned the area, gave me a local anesthetic and then put a lubricated probe into my rectum. He inserted his biopsy gun or probe, with its thin spring loaded needles that would pass through the rectal wall and into the prostate tissue. He told me to expect a little pinch. He should be advised to avoid the words 'little pinch' when dealing with future patients. Each time he took his little pinch from the male gland there was a loud clicking sound, the sound of needles being inserted into my prostate. It felt like he was removing huge chunks, and not tiny samples. I was thankful that they decided not to do a saturation biopsy with about twenty needles. I found the metal rail on the side of the bed and hung on tightly trying to find some interesting pattern in the beige paint. Even a few paintbrush hairs stuck to the wall would have provided a distraction. I could have pretended it was some sort of Rorschach Inkblot Test and diverted myself from the stainless steel attacks at the rear. Unfortunately, they use rollers these days to paint hospital walls and rollers leave nothing but the paint itself to look at.

It has been said that ignorance is bliss. I read that this procedure had no ill effects. There are some temporary ones such as blood in the urine and minor pain, but obviously these are not considered serious. But, my research had me worried about what is called microscopic capsule penetration. The capsule is the membrane that surrounds the prostate gland. As the cancer advances it may extend into this membrane and even beyond. If this occurs the cancer can leak out and attack the pelvis, lymph nodes, rectum, bladder, sex nerves and even the muscles that control urination. By now my dual piss streams were beginning to divide again into three and sometimes four tributaries. Along comes this doctor, and in my imagination, as I stare at the blank wall looking for paintbrush hairs, he starts poking holes in the capsule. Hold on, if it hasn't leaked through, why poke holes in it? I presumed that there is no evidence that it happens. I knew it is not a shell, like an eggshell, but a membrane covering the prostate. But sometimes, as you hold on for dear life and stare at the wall, your imagination can run wild. When he finished removing his samples he turned back to his work area and began filling in his report. I did not ask him about results as I realized they had to be sent off to someone else.

The center of a cell contains most of the material that determines how a cell deals with an attack. It is supposed to defend the ability of the DNA to repair itself. It also should control whether the cells remain in line or go astray. Cancerous cells, under a microscope look like a crab with its legs sticking out. Prostate cells, like all cells, are constantly reproducing and dying. Each new one is the same as the old one, unless cancer cells are being overproduced and not dying. In the case of cancer blood cells, for example, they divide slowly but at the same time, make copies of themselves, which in turn make progenitor cells that do not mature but proliferate quickly and make many new cancer cells. They look different and can be low-grade or high-grade. So the experts know cells can run amok. The real question is why? Why some and not others? Perhaps prostate cancer is spontaneous with many causes. The only way to get a clear picture is through the biopsy.

I started going over my life looking for anything that might have caused my disease. I have done my share of painting, I live in a polluted city, and I have used various products containing Benzene, a known carcinogenic, like shampoos, cosmetics, detergents, cleaners, bug aerosols, fuels and grease. I have cleaned anti-fouling paint off the bottom of the boat without wearing a mask, and used all kinds of plastic containers over the years, and even delivered grimy newspapers as a youth. No one can really say what one, or combination of all these things, might have caused the damage. Probably, and more importantly, I have lived longer than the average man and my group of senior citizens account for about 80% of all new cancers. But this short review also led me to a greater appreciation of the medical staff that work with cancer patients, especially their willingness to expose themselves to even greater dangers.

There was a report, in August 2007, from the B. C. Cancer Agency in Vancouver that a team had discovered the gene, HACE 1 that helps cells to fight off stress and cancer growth. I presume any practical applications are years away.

No doubt some of the forces that open us to cancer are of our own making. At one time in history all disease was seen by some as a result of not trying hard enough to be good. This was especially true when it was cancer of our private parts. Today, we have identified some of the causes, such as smoking, poor dietary habits, pollution, or as one doctor said, just the result of bad luck.

So there I was, facing the bleak wall and the doctor was digging out some cells so that they could be graded and classified. He did not seem interested in answering questions so I remained quiet. At the end I was handed a small typed page that read:

"We need you to stay for one hour. The first 20 minutes to lie down in our stretcher area and rest, and the remainder of the hour to sit in the TV waiting room. If someone is with you, you can sit in the large Prostate Centre waiting area." It went on later to say: "It is unusual to have any trouble after the biopsy, but if you develop fever, increasing pain or any other problem which concerns you, please call your doctor or go to the local hospital emergency department."

I was then led out of the procedure room to a curtained off bed to rest for 20 minutes before getting dressed. I was told to expect blood in my urine and sperm for the next two weeks. He was right about that, well at least in the urine.

One of the results of the biopsy is called a Gleason score and it can indicate how fast any cancer present is growing. The information gathered would help grade the cancer by combining two numbers that add to a total of ten. A pathologist provides results based on the loss of the normal glandular tissue as well as considering shape, size and differentiation from the gland. Scores from 2 to 6 are favorable and a cure most likely. Gleason 7 is considered intermediate and 8 to 10 are considered unfavorable with a low possibility of cure. At the same time it is important to keep in mind that the reading is only for that tiny amount of tissue removed, and will not reveal the whole story. Like everything else these numbers are no guarantee that the score given is exact. However a higher number could mean a more aggressive form of cancer. The extent of the cancer is also defined by the T stage that goes from T1 to M1, the latter meaning bone metastases. I think I came in at a T3b meaning possible extension into the seminal vesicle. By now I realized that at this stage I could never really know just how extensive my cancer was. If the truth were told, I don't think anyone was certain about what was going on at this point in the investigation.

I finally got dressed and met Maureen in the larger waiting room, where we were asked to remain for another thirty minutes. Maureen went off and got me a large coffee and a muffin. I was sure happy she insisted on being with me.

7

On February 8, 2007, we met again with the urologist at the Koffler Centre. As a result of the tests he told us he now believed that there was a thirty percent chance that I had cancer. From fifty percent to thirty percent was a pleasant surprise. Apparently my Gleason score was high, but he did not tell me that, and I should have known to ask. My mind, however, was evaluating the drop in the percentage score. There now seemed to be some hope that the cancer had not moved outside of the prostate in spite of the numerous puncture holes gouged during the TRUS. But what was even more important, after all of these tests, there was still some evidence that I had cancer. This time his pronouncement was not as excruciating as before. He said the usual next step would be a CT scan or MRI scans to determine if the cancer has spread outside the prostate. He then offered us two choices, as we were beyond the point of watchful waiting. I could see he was inviting us into the decision-making process. To make a medical decision about my own body was a serious suggestion, but it was also refreshing to know I was not being told what to do, but asked to take part in the decision-making process.

The first choice he mentioned was a Radical Prostatectomy where the doctor will remove the prostate, surrounding tissue and seminal vesicles. He did not go into any lengthy description of types of Radical Prostatectomy but said it was major surgery. "Equal to a Caesarian?" Maureen asked. Much more serious, was the answer. However I heard that in Sunnyvale, California they have a da Vinci Robot able to pluck the unsuspecting prostate from the body. I did not see any robots lurking around his office.

My second choice was either External Radiation Therapy or Internal Radiation Therapy. External Radiation, as the name suggests, is guided by ultrasound, using a machine outside the body to send radiation toward the cancer. Internal Radiation Therapy, on the other hand, uses a radioactive substance, like seeds, sealed in needles and placed directly into or near the cancer.

The External Radiation Therapy option sounded the least painful and less invasive to me so I blurted out: "I'll take that one please." He gave me a condescending look and said nothing other than repeating the first choice was indeed radical.

I felt totally unprepared to discuss these treatment possibilities. Only later did I realize that he did not expect me to make a decision on the spot. I was so flummoxed, I felt like I had made a fool of myself and appeared very naive. But of course, I was naive. The road we were traveling on was beginning to reveal its many potholes.

He made arrangements for us to consult with a surgeon and a radiation oncologist to discuss these various procedures. It became clear to us that he would not make this critical decision alone. Again, his approach was novel and very new to me. The doctor was not telling me what to do, but sending me out to research for myself prior to any form of treatment.

Later, outside his office, Maureen and I discussed the choices and even considered the possibility that perhaps going to see the surgeon and the radiation oncologist was like going out to buy a new car. Do doctors typically recommend only the treatment they provide? Will each one of them attempt to sell us his or her model? I know at least one patient, faced with multiple choices, who decided to self-medicate using natural products available in any health food store. When I first learned about the enlarged prostate I must confess I did visit a health food store and bought one of the herbal remedies, but felt uncertain about using it and eventually threw it out. This uncertainty made me realize how tied I am to western medical practice.

The urologist arranged for us to meet a surgeon to discuss a possible prostatectomy, or surgical removal of the prostate, as well as a radiation oncologist who would discuss both internal and external radiation therapy. I began to realize that the urologist was some sort of prime director who got things started and then sent us out in various directions to gather information. At least, now I had a better understanding of his role as gatekeeper, the one who knew where to guide us and direct us to the next stage of our journey.

At this time I began to realize just how important was my principal gatekeeper, my GP, or primary care doctor. Without his care I would be blissfully going about my daily life not knowing a serious problem was budding in my body. Dr. James Brooks is my original gatekeeper. Because of all the specialists around today we often overlook the importance of the physician who must start from scratch and get you headed in the right direction. No mean accomplishment. It was his attention to my regular checkups that started me on this unintended journey in the first place. Unfortunately, in Canada roughly over five million people do not have a family doctor. According to one report from the College of Family Physicians of Canada over one million Canadians tried and failed to find a family doctor in 2006 and more than five million people are now without a family doctor. To make matters worse in Canada more than four thousand doctors will be retiring in the next few years. We seem to be heading to a doctor shortage in the future. Those without a GP will end up in an emergency room or a walk-in clinic, often rendering them too late to start proper treatments.

On February 20, 2007, we met with the surgeon. He had before him some of the test results so I was able to ask what my PSA and Gleason scores suggested. I was beginning to learn some of the questions I needed answered. He told us the PSA was low and normal for my age at 4.15ng/mL. On the other hand the Gleason score was high at around 8, at least from where the samples were taken, meaning a more aggressive cancer and a greater chance of spreading outside the prostate. Gleason scores go from 2 to 10, so at 8, mine was considered high with a tendency to grow quickly and spread. But, in spite of the high score, and coupled with a low PSA, he felt there was little evidence of extra capsular extension, or spread of the cancer. Even though he believed it was still confined, he did not think radical prostatectomy was the answer for me. At best, a good medical guess. Trying to determine, for example, if lymphatic metastases has occurred, is critical to planning any future therapy.

A radical prostatectomy does not guarantee that some cancer cells have not escaped and will be found later. At the same time I read that this procedure was not recommended for men over 70 years of age because severe complications can occur. Some of the severe ones listed were: impotence, heart attack, stroke, and blood clots in the legs, infections and even death. Presumably some of these side effects are extreme and hopefully rare. It is also not recommended if the doctors are not sure the cancer is clinically confined to the prostate. His recommendation was high intensity radiation combined with hormone treatment. I told him we had a later appointment with another specialist to discuss radiation. He then arranged for yet another test, a TBBS or Total Body Bone Scan. Prostate cancer often spreads to the pelvic area first and this can happen even if the lumps feel small. Someone wrote on the Request Form for the TBBS under History: "Prostate CA Lymph Nodes." Often cancer can be detected in the lymph nodes as well. He also said his office would arrange for a MRI–Prostate-ER Coil. This is where they place a balloon and inflate it in the rectum as part of the examination. The balloon will allow them to get high quality pictures of the prostate. I was thinking of the The Fifth Dimension song: "Up, Up and Away in My Beautiful Balloon." What will they think of next? With that he grabbed his coat, and left the office. I really did not want a prostatectomy in the first place. I knew of a number of men who had that procedure, only to follow it up with radiation because their cancer had already escaped.

8

Two days later we met with the radiation oncologist in his office at the hospital.

There was a bad snowstorm that day and we were late getting to the appointment. However, when we finally entered his office he was very gracious. Naturally, there was another DRE test. He asked me to remove my lower garments and to climb up on the examination table. Maureen was present in the room so he gently pulled a curtain around the table and explained that someone might suddenly walk into the room. Although it may have been a valid reason, I was happy Maureen did not have to watch him poking his finger up my rectum. Somehow this scene has the making of a good comedy. I asked him why it was done so often, and he said it was very important, as it is helps to determine the stage or extent of the cancer. Staging is the method of establishing the extent and burden of the tumor based on the best available knowledge. I guess the DRE is one of the early staging tools and it does not require any fancy equipment, just a humble finger.

In his opinion, it was still too early to determine a procedure, but he definitely ruled out watchful waiting and did not think radical surgery was necessary or advisable. He was inclined toward external radiation and hormone treatment as the possible procedure to follow. He seemed to agree with the surgeon's conclusions. My frustrated deduction was we were all stumbling around in the dark. But I also realized it was not like removing an appendix or piercing a boil.

The doctor then changed the topic and asked if I would consider being part of a clinical trial rather than receiving the standard treatment.

Trials are research studies that go beyond the standard level of care to find better methods of treatment. At any time, if I should so choose, I could fall back on the standard procedure. Certainly a clinical trial was a treatment option worth considering, not only might it improve my chances, but provide help to others in the future. I said I was willing to consider it, but knowing it was a teaching hospital, I wondered if the word trial was just a synonym for a live body for a new doctor to practice on. God, was I getting cynical. He assured me that he would always remain in charge if we decided to volunteer for the clinical trial.

At this point in time, Maureen and I suddenly realized we had come to the conclusion that external beam radiation was the treatment of choice. External beam radiation is used to give a high dose of radiation to the cancer cells, which divide more rapidly and, at the same time the lowest possible dose to the surrounding, healthy cells. Of course, the prostate is a difficult target because the rectum, the bladder, and the urethra have to somehow be protected. Hence, each program has to be tailor-made to the patient. Intensity Modulated Radiation Therapy (IMRT) uses a CT scan and an MRI to create a three-dimensional picture of the prostate. Computers are used to calculate how to irradiate specific areas while avoiding other areas. They can also adjust the dose to the various targets and help reduce damage. One aspect of this treatment was that it could be done by daily visits to the hospital, meaning life could more or less proceed as normal. Nobody mentioned erectile dysfunction at that point in time, but at my age survival was far more important anyway.

Since doctors really do not know what dose of radiation is the most effective, trying various levels will help find answers. For example, a Standard Radiation Therapy involves 37 treatments and a total dose of 69 Gy. There is a large field of radiation therapy to the pelvis for 25 treatments and a smaller field of radiation to the prostate and seminal vesicles for 12 treatments. In the trial version they will do 42 treatments (another week) for a total dose of 79.8 Gy. They will give a higher dose of radiation to the prostate and lymph nodes and the same or a lower level of radiation to the normal body tissues. The theory is that this approach will cause fewer risks for the patient. I was given an Informed Consent Form and told to take it home and consider it as an option. Maureen and I read the information and I decided, even if it was going to totally screw up my summer of sailing, that I would be part of the trial. I told him I would sign the form. He was a little surprised and even suggested I might want to get another opinion first and suggested Sunnybrook Hospital. I told him I was not interested in another opinion for many reasons, one being it meant I would have to go to the back of the line and start all over again. When the clock starts ticking, wait time takes on a new meaning. You first see the family doctor who arranges an appointment with a specialist, usually off in the future. This is the first long wait. You finally get to see the specialist and he or she recommends a number of tests; this is the second long wait. Finally, you have to arrange another appointment with the specialist to get the results and then arrange treatments, and this is the third long wait. I was not ready to go back and start that journey a second time. I told him that I preferred to find the solution to a problem as soon as possible. So Maureen and I agreed that I should sign the consent form and commit us to the IMRT trial procedure.

It was probably a generic Consent Form that we signed, but there were a few lines that gave me a scare as I read it through. "You are being asked to take part in this study because you have cancer of the prostate. Your cancer is believed to be confined to the prostate gland and the lymph nodes of your pelvis." Were they now telling me it has spread outside the prostate for sure? It went on to say: "It is not known what dose of radiation is the most effective to treat the cancer." In spite of this, I was ready and anxious to get on with it.

It was back in the 1940's and '50's when the University of Saskatchewan started to use radiation for cancer treatment. They used the cobalt-60 machine. Occasionally, in the U.S. the treatment was successful and those who survived were usually the young. Devra Davis in *The Secret History of the War on Cancer* writes about a nurse in the U.S. who described the slow decline many of the patients endured as the treatments progressed. Another therapist said some survived even when repeated treatments burned a hole right through the body from front to the back. Thank God the science has come a long way since then.

"You can usually tell when you are on the right track…it's up hill."
Classic Motivational Quote

No actual treatment dates were discussed at our last meeting with the oncologist and I was wondering when they would begin treating me to more than just samplings of my liquid and body parts. I thought if they found cancer they would want to get right on it. I certainly appreciated the fact that all these procedures were helping to determine the best treatment I required. But at the time, I did not realize what was necessary to prepare a personalized treatment program. I figured they could just book a time and get me started. At that point in the journey I was convinced that I would get only one chance to be treated properly. My anxiety was growing because of the time that it was taking to make these appointments and to gather the information. I was now nine months in the discovery mode and had little idea of the extent of the problem or the possible treatment. Women can make a baby in that time. This was a new experience for me, as I like to tackle a problem as soon as I learn there is one, and then get on with my life. These long delays were beginning to wear me down and I found myself awake at night thinking that my life expectancy was diminishing daily. The longer they put off the treatment, the shorter time I have left. But, I also began to realize it is not a cut and dried process, there are just so many unknowns and the tests and procedures can only provide guiding parameters for the medical professionals involved. Not to mention the interpretation and personal problems the overworked radiation oncologist has to deal with on a daily basis. To make matters even worse, a U.S. newspaper, *The Lebanon Daily News*, commenting on a *Fraser Institute Report* included a quote from The National Center for Policy Analysis: "The Canadian Association of Radiologists says that up to half of all radiology services in Canada ranging from ultrasounds to CAT scans, could be shut down unless outdated and dangerous equipment is replaced immediately." My sense of western medical certainty was being slowly shattered and the world of probabilities was raising its ugly head. Those delays may or may not have had any significant affect on the stage of my disease, but they certainly were having a psychological one, manifesting itself in a lot of anxiety. *The Globe and Mail* claimed that "Radiation oncologists say a wait of no more than two weeks between diagnosis and treatment is recommended. "Meantime, on March 26, 2007, Nova Scotia became the first province to sign on to Ottawa's plan according to a headline stating, "N.S. gets millions from Ottawa to achieve health-care time guarantees. "Accurate staging, or determining how advanced the cancer is, becomes critical to the management of prostate cancer, making long waits between tests very stressful. At what date was I supposed to start counting the weeks?

At the same time I was beginning to wonder who is actually managing my case, the urologist, the surgeon or the radiation oncologist? Or did each of them think the other one was in charge?

Again, in his book *How Doctors Think* Jerome Groopman quotes David M. Eddy, a professor of health policy at Duke University. "Uncertainty creeps into medical practice through every pore. Whether a physician is defining a disease, making a diagnosis, selecting a procedure, observing outcomes, assessing probabilities, assigning preferences, or putting it all together, he is walking on very slippery terrain." Groopman continues: "This is a core reality of the practice of medicine, where in the absence of certitude, decisions must be made."

No wonder they were suggesting after all the consultations that the final decision was left to me. After all, doctors don't like to fail either. On the positive side I felt there was some honesty in admitting there was uncertainty. To me this was better than half-truths or even making important decisions about my health without the maximum amount of information possible. Gestalt, or a fully integrated approach, no doubt has a place, but I was glad, as frustrating as it was, they were taking their time in spite of my rush to get on with it.

The TBBS (bone scan) appointment was on February 26, 2007, and once again we found ourselves in a very crowded and typical waiting room. And wait we did. Two hours later I had the scan and, thank

God, it was painless and, better still, no one asked me to roll over on my left side and raise my knees to my chest. After the scan I asked the technician about the notation regarding the lymph nodes. She simply said, she did not know why that is there. She did not do lymph nodes Then why was it on the Request Form in the first place I wondered? It probably should have been on the request form for the MRI.

However, the MRI was a different story. I definitely got the impression from the oncologist that he considered the MRI important, but he was also interested in a CT scan. In the latter case they would use special x-ray equipment that produces many pictures from inside the body and these images are joined in layers by a computer to give cross sectional views. The Toronto General Hospital has been running tests on a very new and sophisticated, and safer, CT scanner called Aquillion One, but it was not available to the general public. I read there is also another tool called a positron emission tomography or PET scan that can be used for certain other diseases and the best way to pinpoint where the cancer has spread. However, its use is very limited in Ontario and the medical trials are still ongoing. Just my luck.

I subsequently read another article in the *Globe and Mail* referring to the American Medical Association that stated a CT scan can find tiny lung abnormalities, but often missed the fast growing, fatal cancers that can grow between scans. Not my situation, mind you, but something to discuss with the doctor. Whatever approach we were using, notice I said we, we were closing in on some kind of a plan, I hoped.

Now a simple x-ray may provide two or three films for the doctor to examine, but a CT scan can generate hundreds. While providing more information, it also requires more skill to analyze. Experience, I read somewhere, will lead the radiologist to act on first impressions, remembering as well, most of them are hard pressed for time. On the other hand, Duke University Medical Center has a few things to say about the percentage of average diagnostic errors in interpreting medical images. No matter how smart the machine, it's the person who interprets the results that is important.

As soon as I received a date for the MRI I was to inform the oncologist's office.

By early March I heard nothing regarding the MRI appointment. I can understand the delay in getting the actual MRI procedure, but not the delay in setting up the appointment date. Anybody can page through the date book, or computer sheet, and mark in an appointment for the future. I called the oncologist's office to see what could be done. With some asperity I was told it was the surgeon's responsibility. I called the surgeon's office and they said they would look into it.

Ten days later I received a phone call from Medical Imaging Department telling me my appointment was set for, would you believe, almost four months later on June 5, 2007, or one year after I began this journey. I was asked what type of treatment was being considered; did I have a biopsy and when was it performed. I was then told that a MRI could only be performed eight weeks after the biopsy. This was news to me. Perhaps this had something to do with the fact they planned to place a balloon and coil in my rectum and inflate it as part of the process.

Things were still moving more slowly than I was comfortable with. I thought we were off and running after I signed the consent form in the oncologist's office. I used to think wait time had to do with sitting around a doctor's office. Boy, was I wrong. Perhaps, in some parts of the world I would probably have been considering a medical malpractice suit about then. Diagnosis or treatment delayed would certainly qualify for a shot at the big bucks. I sent the appointment information to the oncologist's office as requested.

When the confirmation of the appointment arrived in the mail written in bold lettering across the top was the statement: *** Please note: The MRI scanner operates 7 days a week, 24 hours a day***. But I noticed booking office hours were the usual 9 to 5 Monday to Friday. What about cancellations?

The Fraser Institute's website reported on March 26, 2007, that the wait time for radiation oncology is five weeks. However, if the doctor orders diagnostic or therapeutic technology, there is an additional wait of up to 10.3 weeks. Either there are too many sick people or not enough technology in the Province of Ontario.

2

In the meantime I saw a notice of a talk by a Professor of Medicine at the University of Ottawa. He was presenting his research ideas at the MaRS Centre in Toronto on 'destroying cancer cells with a virus that does not affect normal cells'. It appeared that they were using the Vesicular Stomatitis Virus for that purpose. I emailed the doctor and said I would be interested in becoming involved. I also learned that the Ontario Institute for Cancer Research has an advocacy office. So I emailed them also to see if they could assist me in moving the process along more quickly. I don't know why these organizations give out email addresses, not even an acknowledgement was ever received. Probably scanned out.

Maureen and I attended the lecture anyway and learned it will be many years before that virus treatment, if successful, would become available to the public.

The surgeon's office called me at the end of the month and said they had tried to get the MRI moved to an earlier date. The secretary said the office found the long wait unacceptable. However, since they were unsuccessful I was advised to call the booking office daily to see if there were any cancellations.

I made up a grid to track my calls to the Medical Imaging Department. On the first call I learned that there were no cancellations, and that there were five booking operators who would not mind my calling. I wondered how they determined who would benefit from a cancellation, an emergency or the next person to call? I began calling on a daily basis, except Saturday and Sunday and after 5:00 PM.

In April I lucked out; they found a spot and booked me in for May 23, 2007. Whether advancing the appointment by two weeks would make a difference or not, I did not know. At least it was a start. I asked her to mail me a copy of the change.

On April 3, 2007, I received a call from the oncologist's office. He apologized for the time delay, but said he had been ill and was following up on my case. Perhaps, he was the one in charge after all? He indicated he was concerned about the long wait, and suggested that he book me for a CT scan as soon as possible as my 'pathological profile indicated that we needed to move forward'. What in the hell did that scary statement mean? The appointment was made for the following week. Meantime, I had to pick up a special drink and instructions from the hospital. The CT scan would be done at a hospital a few blocks away from the Princess Margaret Hospital.

On April 11, 2007, we set out for the Toronto Western Hospital, part of the University Health Network, on Bathurst Street. I had ingested the first half of the barium drink the evening before, and drank the other half in the car as we proceeded down the Don Valley Parkway. The pre-drink was provided in a huge paper cup, like a coffee cup, which I attempted to drink between the stop and starts in the early morning traffic. It was slow going and the other drivers probably thought I really liked my coffee. I was instructed to drink the second half one hour before the scan but the drive to the hospital took at least an hour.

As we approached the hospital the traffic was the usual conglomeration in the clogged streets surrounding the building. At first, even though we had left in plenty of time for the appointment, we were unable to find a place to park. We went into the hospital parking lot, only to be waved away by the attendant in his closed kiosk.

We drove down the street toward a large parking garage, but when we arrived, a sign indicated it too was full. Maureen suggested that I get out and go to the hospital and she would find a place to park.

Soon after Maureen arrived and we joined two other people sitting in the waiting area. I picked up a magazine that was as recent as two years old, and began reading an article. Almost at once the attendant came in and asked me to change to the usual hospital gown. I put on the gown, still not knowing if it should be back or front opening, and discovered that there was no place to leave my street clothes, so I carted them down the hall to the procedure room.

The imaging technologist-in-training actually strapped me onto the table. He then commenced reading from a card a list of the potential and terrible things that could happen to me after he injected the colored dye into my veins. I could even have a heart attack, he said. I did not expect red dye, as I thought the awful drink I had in the car coming down was all I had to ingest. He and his supervisor, who then joined us, assured me they were not trying to scare me, but that it was something they had to do even though complications were very rare. Welcome to cover-your-ass medicine.

Finally, after the injection, the machine began to move and I slid into the large doughnut like apparatus. It was over in a few minutes and I was told the procedure was finished. They then gave me a card that said, "Some people can have a reaction to the dye." Among other things, it could cause a red itchy rash for one or two days. If I experienced any of the problems mentioned on the card I was to proceed to the nearest emergency room and show the card to the ER doctor. None of the possible symptoms appeared in the following week.

Although a CT scan has greater risks than a simple x-ray, it provides a much better picture. Computerized Tomography will show the size and shape of any tumors and the location in the body. It can also distinguish whether the tumors, if present, are solid or hollow. The red dye is intended to be a contrast medium to improve the pictures. The radiologist would interpret the results and inform the oncologist.

Dragging my clothes back to the waiting area I got dressed and together we left the hospital for the drive home. The barium drink sat heavy in my stomach. However, since I did not have any food or drink for almost a day, I was anxious to get home.

3

On April 19, 2007, we met with the oncologist for a second visit. He was very generous with his time and willing to discuss our concerns. We appreciated his approach and felt we were finally getting some personal attention.

The question came up again regarding the Clinical Research Study. He said I could still refuse to participate or withdraw from the study at any time. The balance here is quality of life versus quantity of life. I think at that time I was not willing to sacrifice quality for some possible quantity. Brave words when I was a good distance from the edge of the cliff. No doubt here was some sort of trade-off in making that decision. An aggressive approach could have serious impact on the quality of my life, but the clinical trial I agreed to, seemed less aggressive. On the other hand, a conservative approach to treatment, the one I expected, could result in improved quality, but might in the end, shorten survival time. He tried to assure me by pointing out they would use the latest method of treatment called conformal intensity modulated radiation therapy, or IMRT.

The IMRT procedure would go something like this: Three gold markers would be inserted (TRUS again) into my prostate using the special ultrasound machine through my anus. I thought I should buy a magic marker and draw concentric circles around my butt. But at second thought, they did not seem to have any trouble locating the center of their target, the posterior opening of the alimentary canal, my anus.

Speaking of targets, the gold was to provide markers so that the radiation could be directed to the proper place. Before the days of DNA and huge insurance claims, some chemists decided to figure out the value of the human body. So they broke down the elements and compounds and priced each one. The result was a human body was worth $2.32. Adding the value of the proposed new $22 gold deposit, I would be worth $24.32. Finally, I am starting to see some good results!

The oncologist then scheduled another CT scan, and two more MRI's were on order. One MRI was a diagnostic tool and the other was for radiation planning purposes. Again, these were to give the radiation oncologist a better map of the area to assist him in the development of my personal computer program which I now realized was required. The total amount of treatment considered was five days a week for eight and a half weeks. This had to be calculated into the program as well.

He then gave me a prescription for an injection of Lupron Depot PDS (leuprolide). Little did I realize then what a pain in the butt this drug would become later. I was told to bring it to the hospital on April 26 for the injection into my backside. Lupron Depot is a palliative treatment and not a cure for cancer. It is used to reduce the level of male hormones like testosterone, which is produced by the testes. Although testosterone does not cause cancer, most types of prostate cancer need this male testosterone to grow and spread. So androgen deprivation therapy, or ADT can make prostate cancer shrink or slow down but not cure it.

Plain and simple, hormone treatment is a form of castration. The alternative is orchiectomy, or surgical removal of the testicles. Back in the early 40's a Canadian doctor won a Nobel Prize for that particular discovery. Using a drug, developed in the early 80's, seemed a much better alternative to orchiectomy, but with the same results. What I was not sure of at the time was whether this chemical castration was final?

The prostate usually has a lot of responsibilities such as supporting sperm, inhibiting bacterial growth, liquefying spermatic fluid, urinary control and forcing sperm out of the penis. I realized there would be no more teenage fun in the shower once I started the treatment. I knew homo erectus was extinct, but that I would become a homo non-erectus never crossed my mind before. Was getting old some sort of reversal of human evolution? I hoped the drug would not eliminate the designation homo sapiens as well, much as I doubt that label is true.

I was told I would be getting these shots every four months. It looked like my busy little prostate was going to join its owner in retirement. Thank God the Province covers the cost as each shot runs about $1,400. The first injection was scheduled for April 26, 2007. I was provided with a reminder card to bring to the appointment. Perhaps the hormones would dull my memory as well?

As if castration is not bad enough, this drug can produce a number of other little nasty side effects: hot flashes, followed by cold sweats, loss of libido, cognitive problems, loss of muscle mass, shrinking gonads, breast development and belly fat, not to mention cardiovascular disease, diabetes and osteoporosis, to name a few of the pleasures I could look forward to.

They say those men between the ages of forty and fifty-five go through an experience much like menopause in women. It is called andropause, or mid-life crisis, and happens when the production of testosterone, the male hormone, begins to decline. Testosterone Replacement Therapy (TRT) is a bit controversial as there are many nasty side effects.

At my age being emasculated by Androgen Deprivation Therapy was not something I was deeply concerned about. As a Leo I have always had a strong sense of self, and I was determined some fancy drug was not going to change that. On the other hand it has been reported that half of the men on ADT, end up in divorce. Not likely in my case as our marriage does not depend on my ability to get an erection. There is even some evidence that pectin fiber, found in some fruits and bran, and thought to protect against dietary and environmental toxins and carcinogens, could become an alternative to my Lupron Depot shots. Or was this wishful thinking on my part?

He also gave me a prescription to purchase Sandoz Bicalutamide and to take those pills prior to the first injection. This drug is also an anti-androgen and it also interferes with the male sex hormones in the body. Once again there are possible side effects like nausea, diarrhea or feeling weak. The printout listed a cluster of other possibilities that I did not want to think about. I just hoped I would be one of the persons to skip those dire results. I was to start these babies as soon as I got the prescription. One consoling thought then was that most of the testing was behind us and this drug was the beginning of the treatments.

Before we left the appointment I was provided with "The Expanded Prostate Cancer Index Composite" a questionnaire designed to measure Quality of Life issues. I took it home to fill out the twelve pages at my leisure and planned to return it at the next appointment. I did not do it.

Finally, we were given the booklet "What to Do When Receiving Treatment".

4

We arrived at the usual parking garage once again on April 26, 2007, to receive the hormone injection. The same few pigeons were still sitting on the ledge and cooing contentedly. As we drove around the ramps looking for a parking space I thought we must have paid a good part of the attendant's salary in the past few months.

We checked into the reception and after a few minutes of waiting were ushered into the oncologist's examination room expecting him to appear to administer the injection of Lupron Depot. However, his assistant arrived, asked me to lower my shorts, and she proceeded to jab the first needle into my backside. I thought my nipples were getting itchy and my voice was getting higher almost immediately. She also said the doctor wanted me to go ahead with the diagnostic MRI, ordered by the surgeon and scheduled for later that month. Returning home in the car I could still feel a slight pain in my right cheek where she injected the drug.

An article in the *Toronto Star* presented a review of the Princess Margaret Hospital's radiation therapy wing. It is considered to have caught the world's attention because of its revolutionary approach to modern medicine. Approximately 7,500 patients receive radiation there each year and an interdisciplinary team of up to 25 staff handles each case. It would appear that I would be in good hands.

Our first introduction to this Centre was to attend an education session. Our appointment was for May 2, 2007, at 10:30 AM.

When we arrived in the waiting area we were led to a small room with a computer screen. The name over the door was Pre Treatment

Education. After such a positive article in the *Toronto Star* we were doomed to be disappointed. The young lady conducting the session had a very glaring accent that made understanding her next to impossible. I hate these situations because for some reason they make me feel like I am the one not communicating. However, with the use of her simple computer program she attempted to explain how I was to prepare each day for radiation treatment. After many frustrating 'excuse me's' on my part I finally understood I should have empty bowels and a full bladder prior to each treatment. It sounded more like 'the queen's balls are full of blubber'. I was not quite sure but she mentioned something about taking Milk of Magnesia each evening prior to going to bed. Milk of Magnesia is a laxative for temporary constipation. Since I usually don't have a problem in the mornings, I paid little attention to this instruction.

During the presentation both Maureen and I became very frustrated but we decided to push on with our questions in spite of our inability to comprehend the answers. After all, this was supposed to be an education or information session. I asked her what type of machine they would be using. I had read there were the older types like the Ionizing Radiation Machines (x-ray) or Cobalt-60 as well as the newer kind such as the Linear Accelerator. She seemed a little confused; perhaps she could not understand my accent. She finally answered that the machines they used were all equally good. Presuming she was a technologist, I asked if she kept a record of her success rate. I thought anyone managing treatment machines would be interested in what their cure record might be. Again she seemed confused and said she did not keep records. At this point in time the teacher seemed more bewildered and uninformed than the pupils. We finally stopped asking questions.

One word puzzled us for most of the session but we finally figured out she was using the word vacuum but we could not put it in any context. She then provided us with a booklet entitled: *Radiation Therapy to the Prostate Area (Conformal & IMRT)*. When asked if we had any more questions, we both stood up and said no and left the office. Needless to say, I was not only disappointed in the session, but frustrated as well. We returned to the parking garage without saying a word. When we sat down in the car I turned to Maureen and said:

"What do you think?" Maureen was even more frustrated than I. We both agreed it was a colossal waste of time and we still had to pay for parking.

On May 16, 2007, we were back at the hospital again. Someone had called the night before to remind me to follow the usual procedures and take the antivirus (APO-Ciproflox 500 Ciprofloxacin HCL) and the Fleet Enema in preparation for another TRUS and the implantation of the gold markers.

Doing the regular Fleet Enema is not the most exciting way to begin a new day. You get a plastic bottle with some clear liquid containing a sodium solution. They define this clear liquid as a bowel evacuate. I call it a fast introduction to Montezuma's Revenge. The revenge angle is that it is a way for those countries that were previously colonized to get vengeance. Thus you have Gringo Gallop, Aztec Two-step, Delhi Belly, Tokyo Trots and Rangoon Runs depending on where you are traveling.

Fleet Enemas are self-administered and even after a fair bit of practice during the past few months, I still found it difficult to insert the rectal tube. You are supposed to lie on your left side, the knee-chest position, remove the protective cap on the tube and as you slowly guide it into your rectum, point it toward your navel, then squeeze the bottle empty. Pointing it toward your navel is just not as easy as it sounds. Once the bottle is empty, or as empty as you can get it, Montezuma starts urging you to get off the cold floor and onto the pot. But no, hang in there say the instructions and wait for five minutes. It is much more fun having your morning coffee or brushing your teeth before leaving the house in the morning than performing these gymnastics.

The waiting room in the hospital was busy as usual and I had to leave Maureen in the larger waiting room as I moved off to the men's only waiting area. This was the same location where I had the TRUS, the Prostate Ultrasound Room #833. Two other men were there in gowns but no volunteers were present this time, so I sat down and read my book. After about an hour, I went out to the area where Maureen was waiting, and reported my lack of progress. Perhaps the price of gold went up and they could not afford it.

I returned to the men's waiting room and found something to read. The May 16, 2007, *Prostate Cancer Research Foundation of Canada*

Bulletin reported that the National Cancer Institute in the USA examined the link between multivitamin use and the risk of advanced and fatal prostate cancer in close to three thousand men. Although they found there was no link between multivitamins and localized prostate cancer, the article suggested there might be a link where there is a family history of the disease and a long and heavy dose of vitamins. Because I have been taking Centrum Select for a number of years, but do not know of any history in my family, I hoped this finding did not cause my problem. However, it was just another morsel of information to keep me on edge.

Finally, someone came and asked me to change. I slipped into a gown and returned to my chair. Almost at once a doctor came out of the treatment area and said there had been an emergency and that was why my appointment was two hours late. He even went to the outside waiting room and talked to Maureen while I was sitting in the procedure room.

When he returned from his visit with Maureen he entered the treatment room and I found myself once again presenting my butt to the doctor and his assistant. But, before I rolled over to the knee-chest position, I said to the doctor: "I know you are running late. I also know most people have a tendency to rush in order to make up time. I hope that is not part of your plan?" He assured me he would do it right so I rolled over and, once again, had the opportunity to contemplate the painted wall as I held onto the rail for dear life.

He then proceeded to plant the gold markers. I love that word plant, as if the little gold seeds were to eventually produce a whole new crop and make me rich. I was not sure how many he injected into me, as I was too busy studying the paint. However, he told Maureen after the procedure, while I was recovering on a cot, that he had placed three markers in the prostate. I realized after that session I now had two useless testicles and three gold nuggets. Was I richer or poorer?

5

The weekend of May 19, 2007, was a long weekend in Canada and we participated in a Yacht Club Cruise along the Lake Ontario shoreline. It was good to get away from all the procedures, but the weather was cold and windy. We stuck it out for three days, and then returned to our homeport in Scarborough Bluffs.

On May 22, 2007, we returned to the hospital for the scheduled CT scan and the planning MRI. Once again I donned the now familiar hospital gown and climbed up on the CT table.

The team proceeded to adjust the machines, fabricating a pelvic form that would keep my body from moving during the actual radiation sessions. The therapist expanded the blue form under me creating a personal mould of my pelvic area. This mould was to be used for the entire course of treatment. Using the laser beams, they located points on my body, one below the navel, and one on each side of my pelvis. Using a fine sterile needle, the technician made three permanent reference tattoos to mark the spots. I asked for two reef knots and a heart, but I got three very small dots. The three targets, the tattoos, the body form, and the gold markers previously implanted, were to direct the external radiation beams to ensure they would not burn holes in some of the healthy neighbors, or so the theory went.

Yet another MRI followed this procedure. I was equipped with earplugs and three very loud sounds later the deed was done. There is no better way to describe the MRI experience than to say you are placed inside a jackhammer and the earplugs only provide some protection.

From there we went for a couple of x-rays and then we were finally on our way home.

The next day I was back again and this time for the diagnostic MRI the surgeon ordered. This was the original one that I had managed to move a few weeks forward and, although ordered by the surgeon, the oncologist's office advised me to keep the appointment.

I was beginning to realize that each test was more effective in finding out what was going on inside me, but more importantly, providing information for developing my personal radiation plan. The DRE is not very reliable in detecting extra-capsular extension (ECE), i.e., has the cancer spread outside the prostate? The TRUS I had earlier may or may not reveal if the zones outside the prostate, or even if the seminal vesicles have been invaded. Even the CT scan is not that reliable. For example, if a very, very small node of less that 5 mm (millimetres), escapes it probably would not have been detected. So I entered the next stage where the doctors were trying to determine if there had been a great escape. External beam radiotherapy will not be effective, in the long run, if distant lymphates have metastasized.

I performed the usual Fleet Enema prior to going to the hospital and considered myself ready. Once properly gowned and seated in the hall, the doctor came out and asked me if I would consider volunteering for his research study. Ordinarily, as was in my case, it was the PSA and the Gleason scores that moved me slowly along to this point. What his team wanted to find out was whether the coil-type MRI could help to search out prostate cancer with more accuracy and discover what might have been missed by the biopsy. What they planned to do was to insert into my rectum a thin flexible tube called a catheter, or in this case an endorectal coil, surrounded with a balloon, which then would be inflated with water to distend the rectum. Then using an endorectal coil with high-signal-to-noise ratio transmit radio frequencies to get the MR images. The prostate cancer will produce low-intensity signals that would indicate if the cancer has extended outside the capsule. I was not sure I completely understood the process, but, if it would help with the diagnosis, and provide better detection in the future, I agreed and signed the Consent Form.

The first thing the technologist did, once they had me on the MRI table, was to explain the procedure and answer my questions. I was strapped to the table so I could not move. Then the balloon was placed and inflated in the rectum. Alleluia brothers, I am in Purgatory, get ready to open those Pearly Gates. More adjustments, or tweaks as the technologist said, and the process began.

Unlike the ultrasound probe, that I found most discomforting, this probe was to be in place for forty-five minutes. I was given an intravenous injection of Omniscan, a sterile clear, yellowish solution. Part of the process included another transrectal ultrasound-guided biopsy. Someone said it might be a bit uncomfortable. That person obviously never tried it. Uncomfortable is not the word; I felt I was literally being screwed!

This whole procedure took almost two hours, not the 45 minutes promised. The earplugs provided were almost useless and the various loud sounds were just as painful as the probe they shoved up my rectum. The different sounds assaulting my ears were those of a jackhammer, a jet engine, an enormous dentist drill, and a machine gun all in some strange sequence. I believe there must have been some noise induced hearing loss; at least my ears were ringing days later. If my hearing hair cells were damaged they will not grow back. There must have been some sort of trade-off there that I am missing. My advice to future volunteers is to bring your own hearing protection device such as earmuffs that have soft cushions that fit around the ear and a hard outer shell with a headband. Don't rely on the ones the hospital provides.

The first thing I did when I got home that evening was to have a stiff drink of Scotch. All this testing was turning me into an alcoholic.

On May 28, 2007, I received a call informing me that the first CT scan and MRI had to be repeated and asked me to return in two days. In one sense this was disappointing as it just meant more delays in getting the treatment started. On the other hand, it reaffirmed the position that they were being very careful in the planning process.

So on May 30, 2007, we returned for a repeat CT scan and regular MRI. When we arrived and checked in we went to the front desk to let them know we were on time. Once again I was asked to fill out a sheet basically saying there were no metal parts in my body. The technologist we met the first time, came and provided me with a large drink of what appeared to be water, but was some sort of oral contrast. We then had to wait for an hour for the liquid to move through my system.

Fortunately, planning for the usual delay, we brought our own reading material. However, I noticed that Maureen, who had just started Wilbur Smith's new book, *The Quest*, had put the book down and was staring into space. I reached over, touching her arm, and asked her if she was O.K. She looked sad and, I thought the whole long experience was beginning to show. I still think this was part of it, but a recent death in the family was also foremost on her mind.

A few minutes later the nurse returned to say there was a cancellation in the Precision Radiation Therapy Clinical and Research Program Support Room, where the MRI is located, and we could go there and get that done while I was ingesting the lovely drink. So we moved over to another waiting room. I must say; waiting rooms are well named. Finally, the technologist came out and invited us into his den. Once again, I filled out the paper saying I had no mechanical parts. He asked me if I had ever had an MRI before, so much for e-health or the use of electronic medical records. Perhaps the day will come when everything will be on the computer and where staff will have hand-held devices containing all they need to know. No wonder the advocates say moving to this system would save money and costs, at least in my case, time and paper. Finally, I was ready and the MRI was repeated, this time with proper ear covers to deaden the much less intrusive sound I had experienced with the endorectal probe a few days prior.

We returned to the CT waiting room where we had started the day. We soon realized the opportunity to get an earlier MRI did not reduce our waiting time. There were always delays in getting things to go right. Finally, dressed in another skimpy gown, I climbed up on the table. Once the adjustments were made to my pelvic mould, the Radiation Therapists stuck little pasties on my new tattooed spots and into the machine I went. After ten minutes of moving me around, I was backed out and told, once again, to go and empty my bowels. For some reason, that there was matter in my bowels, preventing a clear picture on the scan, made me feel guilty. I was told to go and empty the bowel, but not my bladder. This was an impossible command to fulfill. How do you empty one chamber while keeping the other full? I did my best, but ended up emptying both vessels and had to ask for another tanker of water. This interruption meant I had to step outside and wait for another forty-five minutes. I did not return to the waiting area but took a seat outside in the hallway. There were chairs strung along the opposite wall as well as a few tables containing magazines. I sat, thoughtlessly paging through an old magazine, clad in what must have been a child's gown. Each time I relaxed, my knees would separate and I would expose myself to the passersby, unintentionally of course. As Rhett (Clark Gable) said to Scarlett (Vivien Leigh) in *Gone With the Wind*: "Frankly, my dear, I don't give a damn."

I was trying to preserve some modicum of modesty and I reminded myself that I always had problems donning hospital gowns. Do I tie them in the front or the back? I suppose it depends on what side of the body they want to explore. A few times I was provided with two gowns, one to be worn open in the front, the other open in the back. Even after all this practice, it was still a mystery to me. Apparently, some companies have now designed special types of gowns just for seniors that provide adequate access and still preserve one's dignity. The gown I was wearing in the public hallway that particular day, tied in the front but it barely came together and the ties hardly left room for a knot. The same laundry must also provide services to the kids' hospital across the street.

Meanwhile, Maureen had returned to the sitting area at the other end of the hall. Fortunately, one of the technologists went and told her there had been a problem and I was now sitting on a chair outside the CT room. Maureen came down the corridor clutching a brown bag containing a sandwich, one large chocolate chip cookie and a can of pop. The radiologist said I could eat, since I had nothing since five-thirty in the morning. I ate the cookie and saved the sandwich for the drive home.

Finally, I was summoned back for a repeat of the maneuvers on the table. When they were satisfied with their measurements, I was moved once again into the machine. This time the oncologist was satisfied with the pictures and I was dismissed. I was told they required about five working days before they would call me for the actual radiation.

I carried the food to the car, and on our way home enjoyed a chicken/pear sandwich and a can of Sprite. As it was rush hour, instead of heading for the Don Valley Parkway, Maureen drove me north on Saint George Street, which now cuts through the University of Toronto Campus. The street, strange to say, is named after an exiled French

Royalist who had escaped to England, took the name St. George, and then moved on to Canada where he became rich.

We then drove northeast by way of the back streets. It was a real treat. The trees were now in full bloom. I never realized before the size of the forest that exists within the limits of the city of Toronto. From the air Toronto, with its foliage in full leaf, is a city of trees. In fact there are over three million in the ravines, parks and along the streets. Add to that the millions more on private property and you have what is called an Urban Forest. I know it costs the city a little over twenty-five million dollars to maintain this glorious woodland, but this drive helped me to appreciate that expense. A late May drive, after a difficult day in the hospital, through this beautiful forest, was just the relaxation I dearly needed. Maureen knew precisely what she was doing to ease this part of my unintended journey.

6

On June 7, 2007, I received a call from Princess Margaret Hospital informing me that my radiation treatment would begin on June 21, 2007, at 9:30 AM. The long delays had been working on my mind and I almost despaired of getting on with the full treatment. At times I felt like Diogenes, the eccentric Greek philosopher, clutching his lantern in daytime and searching for the one honest man. In one sense it was good we now had a date, but again this whole process had taken so long. Meantime, I was wondering if the cancer in my body was also waiting for the results of all these tests, or was it charging ahead at its own speed taking advantage of the lengthy marshalling delays of its enemy?

At the same time, some of the side effects of the hormone drugs were beginning to show themselves. In the beginning, the Bicalutamide and the Leuprolide Lupron Depot failed to announce their presence in my system, but within two weeks of starting the drugs, I began experiencing my first hot flashes, immediately followed by cold sweats. The female half of the human race knows all about this, but it is confusing for a lowly male. It was difficult to distinguish between a hot day and a hot flash. This was complicated by the fact it was the springtime when the temperatures tend to fluctuate in Ontario. These episodes averaged about two or three minutes and left my body covered in sweat. I have read that antidepressants have been used and found effective in reducing hot flashes in women, but not much research has been done for men. That is not surprising because it's so unnatural. There is also concern that antidepressants could even support the growth of prostate cancer. Forget that. However, after a few weeks I was able to understand and accept the difference between summer heat and chemical induced sweats. They do say practice makes perfect.

However, when I re-read the literature on Leuprolide provided from the pharmacy, I discovered a number of other possible changes to expect: tiredness, mood changes, occasional dizziness, shrinking of the testicles and reduced sexual interest. I was not sure I liked this chemical manipulation of my bodily functions. I am the guy who would not even take an aspirin for a bad headache. However, I did want to get rid of the cancer, or at least delay its final effect. So I decided at the time, I would bear with the side effects believing they were necessary steps to achieve my final goal: death to all cancer.

During the month of June everything had come to a stop, except the wondering and worrying on my part. It appeared to me that after almost one year of being poked and prodded, drugged and photographed by sophisticated machinery, it was time to begin the treatment. I kept wondering what was taking so long?

Maureen and I discussed letting relatives and friends know I had prostate cancer and we decided it was best to speak about it, provided they in turn, felt free to do so. We knew that the word would gradually get around anyway, especially at the yacht club where we spend a lot of our time with friends. If we were not up front, the elephant in the room would affect the way people treated me. So by being forthright that particular tension was easily dissolved.

In fact, while having a beer one day at the club, the sailors on each side of me confessed that they had been through radiation treatment for prostate cancer and that, as tiresome it might be, they believed their lives were back to normal. This was a consoling and encouraging revelation as I had no idea they had ever silently traveled that road. However, this testimony did not squelch my lingering thought: "Has my cancer escaped from the capsule around the prostate?" It would appear that in their case it had not run away. I now believe that question can only be answered in time, if and when that occurs. Otherwise, no one really knows till it is discovered.

So I was trying to go about my retired life, doing the things I like to do, and talking openly about the cancer within me. But the mood changes and hot flashes just would not let me forget my disease and made me feel as if I were walking across a lake covered with thin ice. I was anxious to get safely to the other shore.

7

It might have seemed frivolous, considering the situation, but I was concerned about getting to the hospital every day. Maureen said she wanted to drive me the first few times. I thought it was an opportunity for her to play some golf, a new hobby she was interested in. With my treatments I would not be dragging her out on the sailboat every day. I suggested that she take a couple of weeks out of town to improve her game, or at least get out frequently to one of the local public golf courses.

Transportation in Toronto is not keeping pace with the growing population and it was a long way from our house to the hospital. One choice was to drive to a parking garage near the hospital as we had been doing for the past year. We spoke to the parking lot attendant and asked if they had a monthly permit for patients. Of course, the answer was a blunt no. There are a number of other lots in the vicinity as well. The Mount Sinai Hospital and The Princess Margaret Hospital lots charge $4.50 an hour to a maximum of $18. The Toronto General Hospital charges $8 an hour and the Hospital for Sick Children charges $7 an hour. If the treatment were to take eight weeks this would be a blow to my budget as our parking bills were averaging $18 a day.

The Princess Margaret Hospital has a lodge at 545 Jarvis Street and a connecting bus. However, it is for cancer patients and their families who come to Toronto from out of town. Since Scarborough, where I live, is not considered out of town, I did not explore the cost. I did realize things had to be kept in perspective, after all, considering the amount of medical assistance I was receiving free of charge, (I did pay my taxes for over fifty years). By comparison, a parking bill was a minor consideration, but it had a very real out-of-pocket consequence.

I could have taken the bus from my home to the Finch Station at the north end of the subway line on Yonge Street, and then proceeded downtown from there. A one-way trip would take about an hour and a half, if things were moving well. Hence, three hours a day on the bus and subway line was not appealing in the summer time, although thousands do it. I had found from experience once on board the subway, with a good book, or engaging in intense people watching, the time can go by profitably and quickly. But I was not ready to make that concession of time.

Parking was just one small, but important problem to solve and I wanted a plan ready to go before starting my treatments. I could have avoided the bus ride to the subway at Finch, and take the car to Fairview Mall to catch the subway there, saving some time. However, all the parking lots at the mall were closed during the morning rush hour making that choice difficult. I decided to visit the Administration Office at the mall to gather some information. The front desk informed me that there was parking for three dollars if you arrive before 9:30 AM. I wandered around this large mall looking for the entrance and the coin machines. I was unable to find them, and, as I re-entered the mall I saw a booth providing information for Community Services. There was a middle-aged woman sitting behind the information counter. She was wearing a long black loose summer dress and wore a broad-rimmed straw hat. She looked approachable so I decided to try there. The lady was very friendly and said she was not sure of the location herself. She turned around to face the back office and said she would be leaving the desk for a short time. She came out into the mall corridor and the two of us walked to where she thought the coin machine was located. However, we soon discovered it had been moved to a new location. After some searching, we finally found it. She was pleased we took the walk together as it gave her information to help others. In spite of what Toronto haters say about our city, in my books, it is still Toronto the Good.

I have been told there are volunteers who drive cancer patients for treatment. That might have been an appealing option, except that in a conversation with one volunteer driver, I was told there are countless delays and long waits at the hospital as patients complete their treatment. This alternative really made me feel I would completely lose control over my life.

Losing control over my daily schedule was probably the second major jolt to my retired lifestyle. After many years as a member of the work force, retirement afforded me the freedom to plan my own use of time. Suddenly, I learned I would no longer have that freedom. Driving everyday to the hospital would be tantamount to a return to work. At least I would not have to wear a shirt and tie, but I might have to consider parting my pubic hair to look presentable to the radiation technologists.

A friend of mine, who had completed radiation a few years ago, said he solved his transportation problems by using his bike. However, he did say he had to stop two or three times on the way home to empty his bladder. A bike was definitely out for me. He lived downtown and not in Scarborough as I do. Remembering the rule, empty bowels and full bladder, I would have had to learn where the restrooms were in the subway stations. Perhaps a monthly pass would be the answer? I would like to think my mind was dwelling on these mundane issues to release me from the negative thinking about having cancer.

Another concern, during this interlude, was the tendency to eat more than usual, and neglect my scheduled visits to the gym. Somehow, the things I had always done to keep in shape began to lose their importance. I did not totally dismiss the idea that my new journey could end in the funeral parlor. Somehow, I had to work around these mental barriers, obviously caused by the drugs, and get back to proper eating and working out.

I tried to spend as much time on our sailboat as possible as I was beginning to realize that if the treatment was delayed any longer, the sailing season would be cut short. I had hoped we could get it done prior to July and August, the best two months we have for sailing on Lake Ontario. Of course, that did not happen.

8

Finally, the day was approaching when the radiation treatment was to begin. But I received a call the Friday before, informing me that the oncologist and his team required even more time to prepare my case. I was informed, with apologies, that the treatment would be postponed for three more days, the new start date being Thursday, June 28, 2007.

Maureen was a bulwark and knew how much I wanted to get started. I had realized by then the sailing season was a write-off. I tried not to exhibit anger, frustration, or discouragement. After all, it was only a simple change of dates, but the disappointment was major. I was so ready mentally to begin this thing, and then had to suffer a further delay. Did that mean they are really doing a good job, or were these delays a result of something else? Somewhere along the line I had planned to discuss the impact of these postponements with the oncologist.

Unfortunately, I had already started taking the required Milk of Magnesia, but it is not a good idea to take a laxative before heading out onto the lake in a small sailboat. Maureen saw the positive side of the delay and suggested we spend a few days cruising. I was not up to that and, in the end, we ruled it out and just moved onto the boat, tied up to the dock and close to the bathroom. It is very difficult to use the small head on the boat when it is heeled over and smacking into large waves. Besides Maureen is much more comfortable if I am on deck while under sail. When I have to leave the cockpit to visit the head, Maureen takes over the wheel. Her first question is always: "What is the compass course?" followed by her admonition: "Don't take too long!"

On June 27, 2007, I was having a cool beer on a friend's boat near our boat slip. It was early in the afternoon. Maureen was at home enjoying a game of bridge with her friends, or so I thought. I glanced over to the parking lot and there she was, dressed in her street clothes, and heading in our direction. She stopped near the end of the finger dock and beckoned me to come over. I got off of the boat and sat down beside her on one of the nearby dock boxes.

She told me the doctor had called earlier when she was out. She called back and he told her that the team would not be going forward tomorrow as planned. Still yet another delay was all I could think. Maureen discussed the situation with him and wisely decided to make an appointment for ten o'clock the next day. I went back to our boat, packed up my things and headed to my truck. I followed Maureen home, a very disappointed person. Delays, delays, delays.

The next day we drove to the now familiar parking garage next to the hospital. As usual it took some time to find a parking space and then to cross over the busy street to the hospital. We announced ourselves and took a seat. Right on time the doctor's assistant came into the waiting area and invited us into the consultation room. Shortly after the doctor appeared. He was very friendly as usual and began talking about the trial treatment and how it differed from the regular one. However, at this point I was no longer interested in the procedure, only interested in getting it started. He sensed my concern and immediately began to explain the reason for so many delays.

He said before they could begin the radiation therapy they needed to ensure a safety zone around the prostate. In other words, it was not enough to have the gold markers, the tattoos and the body form, but it was also important to be sure any damage to surrounding organs was kept at a minimum. The idea was to focus a higher radiation dose to the tumor and, at the same time, minimize damage to surrounding normal tissues. In my case the organs were too close together leaving very little, or no safety zone possible. The team was having difficulty writing the computer program to their satisfaction. Hence the delays. At the same time he pointed out that they discovered 'little fingers of extension' beyond the prostate and possible problems with the lymph nodes as well. *Little fingers of extension* sounded to me like they now believe the cancer has spread beyond the prostate. News I was not happy to hear.

I found the term 'little fingers of extension' interesting. The Greek physician Hippocrates, many centuries ago, described a tumor to be like a crab with its spindly legs extended. He called the tumors *karkinōma*, which is the Greek word for crab. Carcinoma is a malignancy tending to produce death. Those little fingers had a very long history and did not spell good news.

On the other hand, he told me I was in great shape but my cardio-vascular exercise program was creating the problem. They were looking for a safety margin of seven to ten millimetres, and that safety margin was not there. I asked him if this was a usual occurrence and his answer was that my situation was one in a thousand. It became necessary to re-configure the computer program to work within the limits of a three-millimetre safety margin. He had identified the main reason for the delays, and not having a lot of body fat was something I had done to myself.

He informed me that his team had spent countless hours on the case, but had not yet found a final solution. The treatment had to be carefully planned and what they wanted to produce was a custom-tailored radiation dose. They needed to be sure they had those few millimetres as a safety zone. Because of this difficulty they examined various solutions, including surgery, but said that after he consulted with the other doctors, it was decided separating the organs through surgery was not recommended. He suggested July 10, 2007, as a possible start date for the radiation, but I should be prepared for yet another delay if they require more planning. At least now I understood the reason for the many delays and could appreciate their commitment to doing it right the first time. This last visit to the oncologist's office did a lot to restore my confidence in the team I had selected.

After that interesting meeting we went to the blood room and dropped off a few vials of my depleting supply for yet another PSA test. However, the changes, if any, would also measure how quickly, and hence how aggressively, the cancer was growing. Although some doctors do not consider it relevant, there is some research to show that progressively higher PSA velocity readings during the years before diagnosis, along with another risk factor such as a high Gleason score of 7 or more, indicated a greater risk of death from the disease. The key words are 'during the years before diagnosis'. That was when I was having my annual checkups, which always included the PSA test, I think. Nevertheless, I was anxious to hear the latest PSA results.

9

That weekend we went sailing on Sunday afternoon to relax and forget about hospitals and cancer. After a great sail we arrived back and secured our vessel at the dock. Maureen said she was cold and wanted to take a hot shower in the clubhouse. On her way off the boat she asked if I would make a martini and have it ready when she returned.

I had noticed an odor in the boat on Saturday, but thought it was coming from across the waterway where the pump-out station was located. However, on Sunday, the smell persisted and as there were no boats making use of that station, I decided to have a look at our holding tank. Because we sail on Lake Ontario, an inland lake, all pleasure craft must be equipped with a holding tank that is attached to the boat's head or toilet. Each vessel's tank must periodically be emptied into the main sewage system by means of the pump-out station.

The tank on our craft is buried under the settee on the starboard side of the boat. I had to remove the cushions and take away a large piece of plywood, to reveal the tank. I examined the tank carefully and was unable to find any leakage. However, the smell was more persistent. I then decided to remove the teak and holly floorboards and see what lay beneath. Behold, I discovered the source of the smell. The bilge, the lowest point of the boat's hull, contained about three inches of raw sewage.

The previous year I had put in a new toilet and used some hoses that I later learned were not marine quality, i.e., were not high priced. I suspected these might be the problem. However, when I examined the tank hoses everything seemed to be in good working order.

I then decided to remove the hoses and lift out the tank and there it was. The contents were leaking into the bilge water through a small hole in the lowest section of the aluminum tank. What an unbelievable mess. We had been sailing all afternoon in a strong wind, tipping the boat from port to starboard, as we tacked back home. We succeeded in sloshing the contents of the holding tank throughout the bilge area. I procured a bucket and began a very unpleasant task. When Maureen returned to the boat, the martini she requested was not available.

She suddenly decided she would not be staying aboard that night and would go home when the mess was cleaned up. With the help of a friend I managed to get the tank removed from the boat, hosed down the interior and pump it clean. I then washed the inside of the hull with vinegar, dried the boat out with a shop vac and replaced all the furniture and cushions. It was four hours of filthy, grimy work. I wondered if there was any significance with the timing of this event? Was there some hidden message there? By the time I finished, it was me who needed that strong martini, so I too headed home to join Maureen.

The problem with the boat set me off internally once again. I hope I did not manifest the stress I was experiencing but I knew I was ready for a psychological change. I prayed the doctors would be able to clean up my own bilge as efficiently as I had cleaned up the good vessel *SQUALL*.

I was aware, as well, that the hormone treatment I was receiving had a limited time effect. In other words, the cancer cells can adapt and no longer be restrained by hormones alone. So I did not know how long they could put off the radiation treatment.

10

July 4, 2007, may be a big day in the United States but it was another downer for me. The weather was damp and a thick fog enveloped the buildings surrounding our condominium. The fog drifted between the buildings creating a mysterious atmosphere when viewed from our twentieth floor. For some reason this shrouded panoramic view caused me to feel sorry for myself yet again. I tried taking a nap to no avail. I picked up a book I was reading but found it uninteresting. I ate a large lunch hoping it would make me feel better. To make matters worse I was scheduled to crew on a racing boat that evening and the weather forecast was not good. All of this, unusual for me, along with more severe hot sweats and the possibility of yet another delay, incited a feeling of melancholy. Because the sweats and chills required putting on and taking off a wool sweater, the frequency of this forced my mind to constantly fall back on negative thinking. Even though the current Pope had recently said that Limbo no longer existed, I felt I was in Limbo again and very anxious to get some resolution to my problems. This was a new experience for me. Like everyone on earth I have had challenges in my life but I always faced up to them and somehow found a resolution. Now I was being challenged like never before, and yet had no idea what to do, or where to go, other than to stay the course. My hope was still pinned on the oncologist and his team. I believed this to be my best bet. Yet, as I gazed in the mirror my face seemed to have aged significantly, I was tired most of the time, and my interest in my usual activities was beginning to wane. There was an internal sense that

I was confronted with a problem that had no visible solution and it was eating away at my subconscious.

On July 9, 2007, Maureen called the doctor's office to confirm the start date for the radiation therapy. She was informed that the plans had changed again. The team would be using that appointment time to continue fine-tuning their computer program. Hence, I would start the radiation three days later on Wednesday, July 11, 2007.

"I am interested in the future because I intend to spend the rest of my life there."

Charles F. Kettering

Finally, the day to begin the radiation therapy arrived. Maureen drove me to the hospital and as usual finding a parking space in the huge garage was a dangerous experience. We had to drive to the sixth floor before we found an open spot. Entering and exiting cars were speeding around the corners of each floor, and we had to be very careful at each turn. Some of the exiting drivers were swinging in a wide arc leaving little room to pass as we moved up to the next level. Even under those conditions we spotted one or two drivers talking on their cell phones as they one-handed their vehicle around a sharp turn. Finally, after waving to my pigeon friends, we backed into an open spot one floor from roof parking.

We reported at the usual desk located on the first basement level. But this time we were told to go down one floor to the treatment area. Rather than take the elevator we descended the brightly lit stairs that curved around the two lower floors of the foyer. The outside rail is supported by grey steel railings, which are filled with acrylic panels. The arrangement creates a sense you are floating as you descend to the lower basement floor. Tucked around the bottom floor of the atrium, is a beach-like simulation entitled: *Japanese Inspired Dry River*. There are rows of rounded smooth stones, each one carefully leaning against the other. The stones circle between rows of trimmed beech wood. From two floors up, you would expect this rock procession to end in an artificial pool, as it resembled a flowing stream. But the display ends up wandering between the many brown tub-like chairs in the large waiting room corner outside the main treatment area.

Standing at the lowest level and looking up seven floors a skylight was visible. Since the hospital is sixteen floors tall I questioned its authenticity. The next day we decided to check it out and after treatment we took the elevator to the sixteenth floor. The elevator door opened into a bright open area and through the large windows you could see down into the well-like compartment surrounded by the hospital walls. The outside skylight was situated in the middle. Placed around the skylight was the Max Tanenbaum Sculpture Court. At first I thought the figures were skeletons but I quickly realized that the artist, through the clever use of metal strips, created male and female bodies of grace and beauty. There are twenty-five metal inspirational sculptures that can be seen from many of the patient rooms around the court. Many of the patients there were undergoing bone marrow and stem cell transplants and it is hoped they would find emotional courage in the vibrant sculptures that depict such strengths as courage, satisfaction, celebration, creativity and fighting to win. When I first saw this art display I thought perhaps the money could have been put to better use searching for cures for cancer. But, as we studied the beauty of the statues we realized they have a wonderful therapeutic value, even for us. What a great donation to a hospital.

The area where we stood looking down on the statues below opened out into an 8,000 square foot rooftop garden. The floor is made of diamond-shaped panels of a dense Brazilian hardwood. The many planters resemble pillars and are of various heights. The boxes are filled with flowers, herbs, foliage, evergreens and even vegetables. Chain mail, shaped like large flowers and capped with moving antennae, creates a chapel environment. Benches and tables provide seating and were designed to accommodate wheelchairs and hospital beds. The whole place invites peace and contemplation and surely is a refuge for those who find their way there. I was glad I questioned the authenticity of the skylight, as it led me to a wonderful place of peace in the midst of so much suffering.

Meanwhile, back on the bottom floor, the area is called The Samuel Radiation Therapy Centre. A little sign, as you come off the stairs, reads: 'A world leader in the field of radiation therapy' and points out that the ideas of cobalt therapy, staging and computerized radiation therapy were developed there.

I showed my green card with the bar code to the young lady at the nearby desk. She looked at the ID and told me to proceed down the wide bright hall to a much smaller area also furnished with brown leather bucket chairs and several coffee tables. In this area the sign above the reception desk read: Radiation Therapy Reception. The desk attendant got up from her desk and came around the front to show me a scanner, shaped like a small arm. I was instructed to pass my bar code under the scanner, indicating I was Patient-MRN#2626585, present and anxious to get going. At once the screen identified me, indicated that I was scheduled to have my treatment in Unit #4 and said my appointment would be on time.

What a great idea. It would help if all medical offices had something like this. I had been issued the green Radiation Services identification card earlier. My birthday was written on the front, along with telephone numbers for the Switch Board/General Enquiries and the Radiation Therapy Appointment department. More importantly it included my name and patient hospital number. The radiation oncologist was listed as well, and there were lines where I could track my appointment dates and times. However, I did not find it necessary to write in appointment times because at the end of each week the office provided a time sheet. This paper also included a weekly appointment with the oncologist. The card proved to have one serious drawback: I carried it in my wallet where it was a constant reminder that I was a cancer patient.

We took seats in the waiting area. There were a good number of people present, but I also noticed that there were at least eighteen units in operation and the patients moved in and out in an orderly fashion. IMRT is used, not only for prostate cancer, but also for a number of other cancers such as head and neck, breast, thyroid and lung cancer.

Maureen and I settled into the brown leather seats. The other patients were a mixture of male and female. An elderly lady in a wheel chair was quietly talking with two gentlemen. People were constantly walking by; many were staff with ID tags and wearing one of the many colored hospital uniforms of white, purple, green, rust or blue. The patients waiting for prostate cancer treatment were the ones with a bottle of water. They were taking big swigs from time to time in order to have a full bladder and empty bowels as instructed. I dug out my bottle of water and started to drink like the others.

A hospital volunteer came into the area with a tray of fruit drinks and a packet of SUDOKO pages and crossword puzzles providing entertainment for the waiting patients. In one corner of the room there was a basket containing knitting needles and yarn inviting patients, if so inclined and skilled, to add a few rows to a growing shawl. I had no intention of making a mess of that project.

After a few minutes I heard my name called and when I identified myself a radiation technologist trainee asked me to step into the open hallway. She handed us a printed 'Schedule for the Next Ten Days'. She then gave me a quick briefing on what I was to do when she returned later to take me to the treatment room.

We no sooner had settled in our chairs than a nutritionist from the hospital Nutrition Services came along and introduced herself. Maureen asked the oncologist's office to recommend somebody and arrangements were made for us to meet her prior to the first day of treatment. Being on staff she had access to my treatment schedule on her computer. She was able to follow the various treatment changes and delays and miraculously show-up at the right time on the correct day.

We looked for a place to talk, but finally settled into a few chairs not yet occupied by patients, next to the reception desk. There she questioned our eating habits and realized that we were actually doing a fairly good job following the Canadian Food Guide. One item she suggested was a Soy Beverage to replace milk and suggested we might like to try making Tofu fries. I don't like fries of any kind.

We had covered most of the information when the technologist came back to take us to the treatment area. She and another member of the team went over the preparation, such as removing everything below the waist and donning a gown, open in the front of course. I was told I could use the same gown each day for a week. Along with the gown was a clear plastic bag, with my name on it. My pants and underwear went into the bag when I donned the short gown. At the end of the treatment I was to put my gown into the clear container and put it in mail slot #7, ready for the next day.

After I changed Maureen and I were led into the Radiation Room. The area was quite large but the Linear Accelerator occupied a good deal of the space. It generates the photons or x-rays used in IMRT. It appeared to be approximately 10 feet high and 15 feet long. It is not like the CT or the MRI machines that I experienced earlier. There is a metal black table, or bed that moves in and out, or up and down, under the IMRT machine. I climbed onto the bed and was asked to lift myself up as they slid my personal pelvic mould under me. My legs were also placed in a mould-like material to keep them from moving. Shining down from the ceiling were green crossed laser beams. At the head of the table was a large arm holding the linear accelerator, resembling a large saucer that rotates around the table enabling it to deliver the beams at different locations on my body.

The radiation oncology team had set the final computer programs for the treatment. From then on it was in the hands of the technologists. At the end of the second week I was to meet with radiation oncologist. I immediately began collecting questions to ask him.

2

In the IMRT room there were four trained radiation technologists. On the team preparing for this day, but not present were: a medical radiation physicist, a dosimetrist, and somewhere a radiation therapy nurse. Since they are all female, I felt most privileged to have so many young women fussing around my seventy-eight-year old body, searching for my three little tattoo dots.

Maureen watched while I got onto the bed and they prepared me for my first treatment. They lined up the green laser beams with the tattoos, moving me back and forth, until they achieved an exact match. It took a long time to get me ready. I was given a rubber ring to hold as I crossed my arms over my chest. Then Maureen and the technologists left the room. After watching the technologist begin the treatment, Maureen was asked to return to the waiting room.

They began the treatment and the linear accelerator (*Linny!*) started rotating around my body, now and again giving off various buzzing sounds as they applied the radiation. However, what was supposed to take twenty minutes took over an hour. My hands were numb from holding the rubber ring, and my bladder was screaming for relief. From somewhere there was a slight breeze blowing. I did not dare move as they could observe me on their visualizer, stretched out as if I was on display in a funeral parlor. For the sake of modesty I was covered with a thin sheet of paper. But I could feel it blowing around and wondered if they could see more than the graphs on their computers?

Some time later, while sharing the experience with a good friend, he asked: "At what point did you lose your sense of modesty?" It was like asking: "At what age did you lose your virginity?" But if the truth were known I felt like the elderly cynic who said he thought he had gained greater patience, as he grew older, only to discover he no longer gave a shit. I was quickly reaching that same plateau.

When it was over I gathered my things in the plastic bag and hurried to the bathroom where I discovered I had become a mobile fire extinguisher. I got dressed, put my gown in the plastic bag and returned it to mail box # 7.

Day one was now complete and I had a sense of elation that the radiation treatment had actually begun. Of course there were still many unknowns but at least there was comfort in the realization, apart from the drugs to date, a more aggressive treatment had commenced.

The next day my appointment was at 9:20 AM and the process was similar to the first day except it didn't take nearly as long. We had to arise early for the third session on Friday morning in order to get to the hospital for a 7:45 AM appointment. We were the first ones in the waiting area. When I put my card under the scanner it said everything was on time. I was soon called to the change room, but was told it would take a few minutes as they had some preparations to make in the Radiation Room. The procedure went as before, but they had some problems, as I was just over twenty minutes on the bed. At the end I asked a few questions regarding dosage, but the information I was given seemed to be in contradiction to what my doctor indicated. This was the second time an answer to a question did not make much sense to me.

On the way home in the car I jotted down questions for the next Friday meeting with the doctor. I decided no more Milk of Magnesia on the weekend and some R and R on the sailboat. On Monday we were to start again at 12.50 PM.

3

We arrived early for my appointment on Monday afternoon and decided to walk the nearby streets before going into the hospital. Fortunately, we discovered a small parking lot on McCaul Street belonging to Saint Patrick's Church. I went to the office and spoke to the pastor. I posed my problem and he gave me permission to park in the lot across from the church, and even provided me with a sign to put in the windshield. This went a long way in solving my transportation problems, as I was now able to drive down without having to depend on the TTC or pay the catastrophic prices demanded by the large parking lots in the vicinity of the hospitals. However, I would miss the pigeons on the fifth floor. Things were beginning to look up after all.

Even though I was just beginning the treatments I began to experience some mild physical complications. I was told the IMRT was very precise and that the radiation hits the tumor while barely straying outside its perimeters. But it can still do some collateral damage, which may produce incontinence, rectal problems, fatigue and other injury. Each day I was asked if I was experiencing any of those difficulties. I mentioned some fatigue and a burning sensation at the tip of my penis. One of the technologists suggested I drink cranberry juice and not drink alcohol. I have never been a big drinker, but a nice brown, cold beer on a Friday night goes down rather well. Thank God it was not wintertime or I would have been forced to sit by the fire sipping tea. That image does not fit into any of my fantasies of what to do on a cold winter night in Canada.

Of course I did not mention impotence as a problem as I understood it was a result of the hormone treatment. Actually my chemical castration was a sort of bonus, as it prevented anything untoward happening as the bevy of pretty young women pushed and shoved my naked bottom around on the Linear Accelerator bed.

Once the daily routine was established, Maureen decided it was no longer necessary to accompany me each day to the hospital. Rather, she thought once a week would suffice, and suggested it be the day we consulted with our doctor. I felt like the kid heading for school for the first time on my own. I missed her company, but I did not want to spoil her summer fun. Since I was not dragging her off on long sailing trips that summer, the situation provided a splendid opportunity for her to get out on the golf course and improve her game.

I followed the route that Maureen established when she chauffeured me to the hospital. Because my '94 Explorer no longer enjoyed air-conditioning, Maureen insisted in the beginning, that we travel in her car. Now that I was on my own, and the summer weather was upon us, I not only missed our conversations as we waited in traffic, but her air-conditioned car as well.

Facing the early morning drive on the Don Valley was an old experience made new again. When I was working, over twelve years ago, I had to face the rush hour each day on Highway 401. When I retired I figured those days were over. Suddenly I found myself once more, confronting traffic jams and slowdowns, hoping I would not be late for my appointment. Sitting on a hot leather seat, and breathing the carbon dioxide-filled air, was a long way from the sailboat out on the cool lake. Getting prostate cancer is the pits.

One thing I remembered and experienced again was the erratic flow of the traffic. It only takes a parked police car, a stalled vehicle, or an accident to slow down the traffic to a crawl, often just to accommodate rubberneckers. These distractions seem to cause waves long after the incident was gone. The lanes of traffic moved quickly and then suddenly came to a crawl, or even a stop. There apparently is no explanation as a few seconds later the traffic would speed up again. I surmised that the problem was once one car slows down, all the cars behind slow down. When that car speeds up, individually each car does the same thing in turn. Because there is such a long line of cars, with more being constantly added, a stop-start process is initiated and passes down the line, creating pockets or waves along the way long after the original cause was gone.

Part of my journey took me along Carleton Street in mid-Toronto and an area known as Cabbagetown. Even in the early morning that street was bustling with activity and the streetcars were packed with people heading to work.

Two hundred years ago the area was nothing but cottages along the Don River. After the railroad came through, it became a center for Anglo-Celtic immigrants of the Victorian Age. But as these workers moved up the social ladder, the area became a slum. It was rumored that the quarter was filled with Polish immigrants too poor to eat anything but cabbages. Hence the moniker: Cabbagetown. But history shows the area got its name from the Irish immigrants who always had their little plots of land to grow fresh vegetables near their home.

After the Second World War part of the area was bull-dozed to build a housing development called Regent Park Housing. Unfortunately, after many years the area became known for drugs and crime. Recently, the city decided to renovate and a number of families were relocated. Ten acres, of the sixty-nine-acre site, were demolished and a mixed community is planned for the future. It is a twelve-year project that will affect twelve thousand people. Some of the new buildings will be condominiums sold at market value, and others will be subsidized rental units. The question remains: Will people buy the condominiums in an area that is still marked with crime? Only time will tell if this second experiment will succeed.

Many of the old Victorian homes still remain on Carleton Street and a good number of them are in the process of being restored. I saw some symbolism during this daily drive through the old town. Just as the city attempts to restore itself, the medical staff at Princess Margaret Hospital was hoping to add new life to my aging infrastructure as well.

4

One day there were problems with the #4 Linear Accelerator, and, after some delay, I was moved to Unit #3 where there was a new Master of Ceremonies. However, a technologist from Unit #4 was on hand providing some sense of continuity. Along with the equipment problems there were further delays with getting me lined up on the table. The delays, I soon realized were putting a strain on my topped-up water system. My predominant thought, as I lay on the bed under Linny, was the location of the nearest restroom. I even started to worry that I might find it occupied. I could not avoid a few groans, as I lay motionless on the bed.

They say radiation is not painful. This may be true of the treatment per se. However, when you are holding water for a long period of time, keeping it under control, with damaged muscles, it becomes a very painful exercise. When I was finally free, my worst nightmare became a reality. The nearby toilets were occupied. I grabbed someone dressed in hospital scrubs and had her open the employee's private toilet. Oh, what a relief it was, heaven does exist after all.

My appointment sheet indicated that I was to meet a different doctor after my treatment on Friday. I had no idea who he was and why I was not meeting with my regular doctor. I searched around on the Internet and found the blurb for the new doctor and discovered his specialty was DNA Repair and Cell Cycle Checkpoints. Perhaps he wanted to examine my mammalian cell senses DNA double-strand breaks, or something? So I decided to call his office and find out why I was to see him. His assistant did not seem to know and suggested he may be replacing my oncologist who might have been away. Later she called to tell me that was the situation.

So the next day after treatment Maureen and I went to see the new doctor in his office located on the fourth floor. We were soon called into the examination room only to be visited by a female Internist. We never did see the original substitute doctor, so I guess my Cell Cycle Checkpoints checked out.

Her primary interest was the side effects initiated by the radiation. She approved my return to Flomax CR to deal with the numerous night visits and suggested a procedure called a Sitz bath for damage to the anus. I had no idea what a Sitz bath was and ignored the advice. Maureen and I did not like the way she kept looking at her watch leaving us with the impression she had far more important things to be doing. For the second time in this journey we felt a strong lack of communication leading to a sense of vulnerability on our part. I thought I should recommend the book: *How Doctors Think,* but put our first visit down to her inexperience and held my tongue.

A good many years ago I experienced a bad fall while sailing the New York coastline of Lake Ontario. I did some serious damage to my middle finger on my right hand. Because I was out of the country I did not have the injury properly treated and many months later it was necessary to have an operation at a Toronto hospital. Since the doctors used a block, I was awake during the procedure. When it was over I thanked the operating room staff for their help and specifically thanked the principal surgeon using his first name.

When I was being wheeled out of the operating room and down the corridor, the orderly stopped the gurney, came along side and said: "We don't call doctors by their first name in this hospital." I replied: "I am a senior citizen, I will call them anything I like." And with that, and in a huff, he wheeled me to my room.

As someone who was involved in education all my life I understand the importance of maintaining boundaries. At the beginning of the summer semester, I would include a recommendation to faculty not to remain alone after class to assist a young female student. I suggested they step into the hall for any necessary consultations. Often the clothing young women wear in the hot summer months is very revealing and the professor is vulnerable, even to possible false accusations of an unhappy student.

There is no doubt that a doctor, like a professor, is in a position of power. It was pointed out in an article published by the College of Physicians and Surgeons of Ontario: "When you go to the doctor, it's like being in a play, where only the doctor has the script. I know what the scene is about. But the patient is without a script. He or she feels open and vulnerable, and has to rely on others for cues on how to act."

He goes on to point out some examples of crossing boundaries would be giving or receiving inappropriate gifts, providing care in a social setting, not charging for services where you would usually do so, and the oldest taboo of all, sexual contact with the patient.

Since communications are extremely important in the doctor-patient relationship I have found that titles, be they Mr., Mrs. or Doctor highlight the position of power and can impede open dialogue. Hence, I use the title the first few times, but I am more comfortable on a first name basis. This in no way destroys the professionalism of the relationship, but tends to balance the power structure.

Finally, another weekend and we were off for a two-day club cruise to Queen City Yacht Club in Toronto. The weather was great, but the winds were light both days.

On Monday afternoon we were back at the hospital for the next treatment. Once again there was a change in staff and a young man seemed to be the team leader on this occasion. I had been trying to remember names, but I was warned in the beginning by one of the radiation technologists, that they would be changing often. All went well and we then proceeded to the next floor to meet with the oncologist. He was his usual friendly self and once again was very helpful and patient with our numerous questions.

I explained some of the side effects I was experiencing and he said he was surprised and disappointed they were that strong and appeared so soon in the treatment. I explained that I was up often during the night and, only after much effort, was I able to produce a urine flow. However, when it did come, it felt like molten lead running the length of my penis and burning the end as it dribbled into the bowl. He asked if the resumption of Flomax was any help. I said it was too soon to tell, but did not tell him I forgot to take it on Saturday night. Now I was the dishonest one. I planned to dangle that end of my anatomy in the Sitz bath and hoped that would soothe that problem as well. Maureen asked him if the side effects would continue to get worse and he said he would not let that happen. He also said I could start taking my Calcium Carbonate 1250 mg plus Vitamin D again and that they would be prescribing more later.

I was interested in his response to a quote I found in a *Faculty Information* brochure: "Clinical radio resistance continues to be a problem for many patients as a large portion of patients die each year solely from the failure of radical radiotherapy to control the primary tumor." I did not like the words 'many' and 'large portion' and read the statement to the doctor. He did not try to hide anything and said the statement was absolutely true. Some unknowns remained and would do so even after the treatments were complete. This created much ambiguity in my feelings. On the one hand I was not sure I had emotionally come to grips with the grim reality that I had cancer. This alone was a depressing thought. I have seen so many friends gradually destroyed fighting this strange disease. On the other hand, there was reason for hope. Prostate cancer, as long as it is contained, can be controlled. So my emotions sat somewhere between hope and despair when I realized it would be some time, if ever, before I would know the answer. Ultimately, I realized I would probably never stop worrying, for I will never be 100% sure the cancer is gone.

I was aware that the medical help I was receiving was doing some damage to healthy organs. Even the hormone treatment could have some ill effects on the bones, for example. So it must be difficult for doctors to find a balance between healing the patient and causing too much damage in the process. So, even if they were able to contain my cancer, what long-term results might I have to live with after all this exposure to radiation?

A report entitled: *Canadian Adverse Events Study* pointed out that one in thirteen Canadians is harmed by the medical care that is supposed to help them. *The Fifth Estate*, a TV program, did a documentary entitled "First, Do No Harm." The actual words of Hippocrates in *Epidemic* ('On-People') were: "As to disease, make a habit of two things – to help, or at least, to do no harm." But with modern medicine, at least the program I was in, part of the healing process is actually to do some harm. How this differs from the *Canadian Adverse Events Study* is that the harm is intended and unavoidable, and not the result of ignorance and malpractice. The greater good is the goal.

5

I was getting to know the staff in Unit #4. There was usually a change of one or two now and again, but there emerged a nuclear group. Each morning they ask my birthday to establish identity. However, on the Friday that actually was my birthday, they did not ask for that ID and proceeded with the radiation. On a previous occasion when they forgot to ask the birthday question, they went to my file and looked at my picture. So I thought that was what they were doing this time as well.

When they were done and the bed was being lowered, their voices came over the intercom singing the Happy Birthday song. I was deeply moved. They explained they did not ask my birthday prior to the treatment in order to surprise me at the end. It was great and made me feel I am not just #2626585 to them, but a real live person.

Besides Maureen, there were still a few people out there who loved me; at least judging from the number of Birthday cards in the mail. One from my brother said on the outside: "Another Birthday and you still look great." On the inside of the card there was a large chimp with a huge grin and waving his arm. My brother wrote: "Hope you get rid of the 10 ton gorilla cancer. No need to keep it. You can get on fine without it." Another card from a dear friend had the word 'HUG' seven times on the outside, and inside "There's a hug for each day of the week!" Still another, from a couple of friends from the yacht club read: "On the highway of life, there are bound to be some bumps in the road along with crater-sized potholes, backed-up construction traffic and that one jerk who always cuts you off. But anyway, you'll get through it." It's surprising how the little things in life meant so much, even when those damn hormones were destroying my manhood.

Maureen always set the alarm clock to be sure we were up and ready for the hospital run. I hate alarm clocks, as the sudden noise is so harsh there is not time to adjust to the new day. I like to wake slowly, locate myself on the planet, and even listen to some music in bed before letting the bare feet touch the cold floor. On the other hand, I am glad she set it just in case my internal clock let me down. Usually, my bladder bell goes off long before the clock. So when I wake up, I turn the clock off before it rings and get Maureen up with a steaming cup of hot coffee.

On Monday Maureen drove me to our new parking place near the church and we walked over to the hospital. It was a hot summer day but a slight breeze, and the shade of the tall buildings, made it quite bearable.

Maureen left me at the foot of the stairs near the Japanese River and I went on down the hall to check in with my bar code. Because the traffic was light we were an hour early for the appointment. I had no sooner settled down to read my book when a technologist poked her head around the corner and asked if I had taken my litre of water? Unfortunately, I had just finished drinking it and so missed an opportunity to get treated early. There was yet another new technologist on duty standing by the Linear Accelerator who informed me that she would be part of the team that week.

There was one mishap with the body form. They seemed to be having all kinds of problems getting the laser beams lined up and were pushing me back and forth on the table. Finally, they noticed that they had placed some other guy's body cast under me. I had to get up while they produced my personal mould. After that adjustment, lining up the targets was a success.

At the end of the treatment we went up one floor to meet again with the oncologist. There is no doubt he was keeping a sharp eye on my progress. We were there a few minutes when his assistant came along and said we should have checked in at the reception desk on that floor as well. I said I used my bar code ID earlier. In spite of the impressive technology, she told me I also had to report on this floor prior to each meeting with the doctor. Probably has something to do with OHIP?

As I wandered down to the desk I could not but help notice the number of people waiting in the area near the education rooms. I realized many of them were at the very beginning of a long journey. Most of them were there to participate in the Education Program or to get fitted with the tattoos and body moulds. In a sense I felt like a veteran as I passed through the area, after checking in, and moved further down the hall to the treatment rooms in search of the oncologist's assistant.

This raised an interesting thought. In spite of all the effort to inform the patient there still lingers the notion that something is missing in this process. It is like any form of learning, you hear the instructions, you read the literature, but you really don't understand what is going on till you actually submit to the process. I have found that it is only after I have traveled down a road that the printed material begins to take on a new and more powerful meaning. So these future candidates for radiation were probably bewildered, as we were, in spite of all the hospital's effort to eliminate misinformation.

We only had to wait a few minutes when we were ushered into a treatment room. Soon the internist appeared again, this time dressed in her white coat and stethoscope. She seemed much more friendly and relaxed since our last session two weeks prior.

Again she informed us that she was there to answer our questions. I regurgitated the burning penis and the vice-like rectum syndrome, burning like a Ring of Fire, to quote Johnny Cash. I asked if these conditions were a form of cystitis and procititis. She answered that radiation causes irritation not inflammation. This did make some kind of sense about what was going on. I presumed then that the radiation is an irritant, or an external source, making the bowel and bladder uncomfortable. On the other hand inflammation is a protective attempt by the body itself to remove a stimuli and to heal the tissue. She again recommended the Sitz bath. I decided I had better take that recommendation seriously this time. I found out the name Sitz comes from the German word *sitzen*, meaning sit. It is often recommended to ease the discomfort from infection, painful ovaries, or vaginal pain. Since I was not experiencing any problem with my ovaries or vagina, I guess she was thinking of my anus. Once again I did not bring up the hot flashes, chills and bouts of fatigue that were daily occurrences. Perhaps they will be recommending a training bra next?

The instruction sheet I received at the hospital regarding the Sitz bath suggested using the bathtub for the treatment. Then it went on to say: "dry the bottom by patting the area with a clean towel or use a blow dryer set low or a hand-held fan. " I thought this sounded rather kinky and might even be worth a try.

Poor male that I am, I presumed that the Sitz bath was some sort of prescription that I had to bring to the pharmacist. The next day I asked the ladies in the radiation room and they said a prescription was not necessary and left it at that. So, after returning home, I went to my local drugstore and searched up and down the aisles looking for a packaged Sitz bath. Not finding anything I turned to the druggist for help. The pharmacist, with a strange smirk on her face, said I could purchase it next door at the local grocery store. The product to be used in the Sitz bath is Sodium Bicarbonate, good old $NaHCO_3$. I wanted to hide behind the nearest counter display. I was requesting a prescription for Cow Brand Baking Soda. I wonder if the Ontario Health Plan would cover it if I did manage a prescription? That evening Maureen presented me with a *bain de siege en plastique* – a plastic Sitz bath that fits on the toilet bowel when the seat is up. Of course, like everything else, it was made in China. At least I don't have to clean the bathtub after each session.

6

The rest of the week went well and I was looking forward to the long weekend. Ontario celebrates Lord Simcoe Day in early August. John Graves Simcoe was the first lieutenant governor of Upper Canada from 1791 to 1796.

John Simcoe introduced courts, trial by jury, English common law and even more importantly abolished slavery, long before England did so. An interesting part of his history was the construction of Yonge Street running north-south and Dundas Street running east-west. Even in those days these streets were not in the best of condition and were often covered in mud. He modeled them on the military roads built by the Romans when they occupied England. He intended to use them to aid in the defense of what was then Upper Canada. I wonder what he would think if he could look down today on the town dubbed Muddy York?

I was happy to have a few days off from radiation and went down to the boat early Friday afternoon. Saturday was a beautiful, but hot day, and I was invited to motor out and anchor off the beach for a swim. The water was refreshing and rejuvenating. On Sunday, my niece Ann and two friends came down to the club and we were off for a terrific sail. The wind was about ten knots when we started out, but it picked up to fifteen and twenty knots later in the day. With the boat's rail in the water we gave the kids a thrill and then returned to the dock for a lunch of sandwiches provided by Ann and her friends. I had a choice of lobster, chicken or a roast beef sandwich. I happen to be a lobsterman. The sandwiches were followed by home made cookies and then, a long walk to the lighthouse situated at the Bluffers Park harbor entrance. It was another hot day and the park and beach were crowded with picnickers and swimmers. As we dodged through the various groups we could smell the delicious ethnic dishes cooking on the portable stoves.

Although Monday, the actual Lord Simcoe holiday, proved to be another beautiful day, I had pushed myself too hard the previous day and needed to rest. I spent most of the day reading in the shady cockpit, dozing, or just watching the many pleasure craft moving in and out of the harbor. However, I was learning that rest alone does not solve the problem of fatigue. The radiation treatment, coupled with the loss of sleep because of the frequent nightly travels to the bathroom, were the source of my lethargy. Just resting, although necessary, did not eliminate the feeling of exhaustion.

Tuesday morning I was back to work. Some of the regulars were there to welcome me to the treatment room. Once on the Accelerator Bed with my friend Linny, they were able to mechanically move it up and down or back and forth. They also would move me a millimetre or so by reaching across my body, grasping both sides of my gown, and giving a jerk one way or the other. These adjustments were necessary to line me up with the various markers as indicated on the nearby computer screen. On this occasion they asked me to lift up my body to adjust the pelvic mould. While lifting myself on my elbows and heels, my right arm slipped off the bed, and I crashed down on the table before they could reinsert the mould. There was no damage, but the noise was so loud I thought I had smashed the glass top. I should point out that in spite of all this shoving, moving and adjusting, it was often still necessary to stop the treatment, have the staff return to the radiation area, for one final adjustment of the bed.

Halfway through that day's session, they announced on the PA that they were still having a problem with the computer equipment and there would be a short delay. No one told me my crashing down earlier had anything to do with the malfunction. Five minutes later they came into the radiation room and lowered my bed and told me to take a break. I pointed out that my bladder was in no condition for a delay of any length of time. We all agreed a partial spilling of the bladder was impossible. So I rushed to the bathroom, and then quickly recharged my bladder by gulping another jug of water. While I waited in the hall, I watched the technician work on the computers. There were about six or eight different screens spread out on a large angular countertop. Summoning up my courage I ventured into the control area of Unit #4 to find out what was going on. I was told there was a problem with a modem. As a result the multileaf collimator (MLC), which provides conformal shaping of the treatment beams, was down. By moving independently of the radiation beam the collimator will block or protect the healthy areas around the tumor. What I saw on the screen were red borders. The red borders should converge on a particular mapped area of my body plan, adjusting the size and shape of the computer-determined radiation beams. One border refused to move. These red margins are supposed to come across the screen and surround the selected zone. In this case, because of a modem malfunction, one frame refused to move. Hence, the machine locked up and the treatment stopped. A neat safety factor to protect my healthy parts.

Intensity modulated radiation therapy (IMRT) uses beamlets, or very small shafts of radiation, and aims them at the tumor from different angles. Hence, it was important to position me just so on the table. The intensity of each beam is controlled and they can change the shape hundreds of times during the treatment. As the Linear Accelerator rotates around my bed-table I could hear it focus on the target and then begin the radiation beam. To me it sounded like they first load the gun and then fire it. So when the therapists would leave the room I usually said something like: "Happy shooting, ladies." Later I learned the proper terminology was 'Step and Shoot'.

These beams can actually change shape in order to avoid healthy tissues. That is why the preparation period took so many weeks for the team to accurately define my unique parameters. All the MRI's, PET and CT scans, x-rays, gold markers and tattoos were part of defining my personal plan. That day was the first time I had a chance to get into the control room and look at some of the computer screens.

The repairman was moving back and forth between the control room and the Linear Accelerator. As he passed me standing there in my gown I said, tongue in cheek: "I'm sorry I broke your machine." He responded: "Oh no, it is not your fault." No sense of humor but, more importantly, an indication he understood the seriousness of his job. Fixing one of these machines means more than just bad information spitting out of a printer; mistakes could affect the health and even the life of one of the patients or staff.

Up until now I thought there was an actual window somewhere where the radiation technologists could keep an eye on me. I tried, on occasion to roll my eyes around hoping to get a glimpse of them peering out at my half naked body. Previously, when I had the simulation test and the tattoos scratched onto my body, there was a glass window with curtains, and I could see the staff in semi-darkness looking at their computer screens. I soon realized that in Unit #4 there was no window. How then did they keep an eye on me? When I was in the control room I asked about the window. She showed me two monitors that gave an excellent view of the Linear Accelerator and, when I am stretched out on the bed-table, of me. They could also speak and listen to me if need be. I guess you might call it a modern window. I was being watched, up close and personal, on TV.

Finally we were back in business and they had to line me up once again. No sooner than we started, the machine broke down a second time. Thank God I voided my bladder earlier. Finally, things were finished and they came into the radiation room to set me free.

As I got off the table I told the technologist that when under stress I usually try to visualize a comfort zone. My regular fantasy zone is a tall shady tree, surrounded by lush green grass. I am lounging under the tree on a warm sunny day. To add to the exercise I usually add sound, the sound of the water trickling down a nearby creek. Not a good fantasy when your bladder is in need of immediate relief.

The next day when I went into the Radiation Room I walked up to the Linear Accelerator, which I now regularly address as Linny, and told it I was sorry and asked it to behave properly. Guess what? It worked! The machine and I were actually beginning to make friends.

7

When I was a small boy I found a baby robin that had fallen out of the nest. I took the tiny bird home, made a little home for it in a box with a grass nest. I fed it often with an eyedropper. Each time I squirted some food into its gaping beak, something popped out of the other end. At this stage in my treatment I was beginning to respond to food and drink in the same way. After a meal, or even a snack, I was off and running to the nearest bathroom. All of this exercise resulted in a sore bum. The Sitz bath is supposed to take care of that end, but I had to take the treatment four or five times a day. I was beginning to learn that treating prostate cancer is a truly a full-time job.

One day I decided to count the number of times the Linear Accelerator turned and how long each shot of radiation lasted. There were about ten different locations and the duration of the radiation varied each time. After the treatment I asked about it. In the course of the conversation I was informed that they would be starting a different routine very soon and the rotations would also be a different sequence.

That same day we had a meeting with the oncologist. As usual he was most pleasant and created the impression, even though he is very busy, that he had all the time in the world. I did not wish to take advantage of his openness, but at the same time I needed to know what was happening to my body.

Although they were unable to tell if the tumors were shrinking, he did emphasize the fact that the earlier treatments were providing mostly prophylactic coverage to the pelvis and lymph nodes and less to the prostate itself. However, with the change of venue, as the technologist had recently pointed out, I could expect a higher dosage to the prostate proper.

I was curious about success and wondered if there was a way to tell how the treatment was progressing. Hence, I asked him when they planned to do another PSA test. Patients who have a lower PSA score after the radiation is complete usually are less likely to have their cancer return or spread to other parts of the body. But what about during the treatment? If they did a PSA at that time could they get some idea how well I was doing? Unfortunately, the answer to that question was no. During the early weeks of treatment, PSA levels usually rise steeply because the radiation elevates the PSA serum levels. Hence, any measurement is of no value. They will only measure the PSA three to six months after the radiation is completed. I read somewhere that with a patient receiving 1.8 Gy each time, the PSA tends to slope after four weeks. In my mind at least, it was a valuable question.

As to my question about fatigue, he said it was due partly to the hormone treatment and the radiation and agreed it was also because of my many night visits to the bathroom. The frequent trips interrupted my sleep patterns and the body did not like that change. I told him gleefully that I woke up one morning with a partial erection. He deflated the situation by saying it was not a normal erection but simply the result of poor positioning during the night. That ended that dream.

On the matter of frequent bowel movements, not diarrhea, he suggested a better control through diet. He said I needed to establish a very bland diet and abandon a healthy diet of lean meat, grains, fresh fruit etc. As we left his office we asked to see a dietitian again. His assistant arranged for a visit with a dietitian that same morning.

In practice I had to choose grain products made with white flour, eat fewer fruits and vegetables, eat lean meats and drink lactic acid free products. Worst of all, I had to avoid caffeine and spices. The dietitian even gave us a sample meal plan, a plan I guarantee will not appear in the *LCBO Food & Drink* magazine in the near future.

The weekends were a great relief. Friday night and Saturday were becoming the worst days of the week, due to exhaustion. By Sunday I was beginning to recover and by Monday, when feeling much better, I was back in the 'step and shoot gallery'.

We went to meet with my doctor after another treatment. We climbed up one flight of stairs and I reported to the desk situated on that floor. We were directed down the long, but now familiar hall, and took a seat on the chairs lining the wall once again. His assistant came along quickly and guided us into one of the treatment rooms. Again the internist appeared but was more relaxed this time. We had a few questions for her regarding PSA measures after the end of the treatment. I guess I am no different from anyone else, as I wanted to know how I was doing? The oncologist had made it clear they cannot answer that question until some time after the treatments were complete. But I thought I would hear what she had to say anyway. Dead cancer cells are gradually dispersed from the body and some, even though technically dead (meaning they cannot multiply) may hang around for some time before they die. PSA levels may culminate after the first four weeks of treatment, but it takes a long time to get an accurate reading indicating the results of the radiation treatment.

After she answered our questions we were taken into another office and shown the computer programs used for my treatments. Including the radiation oncologist there were three doctors in the room with us observing the demonstration. The display included my x-ray type images with the computer measurements applied over the top. Maureen had requested this on Friday and he lived up to his word. We gathered around a computer screen and saw where the gold markers had been placed, the tight organ space they had to work in, and some of the planning procedures that went into setting up my program. The Linear Accelerator will not deliver a higher dose than prescribed and it will not even turn on until all the treatment requirements are perfect. It is checked each day with a piece of equipment called the Tracker, or a class of software with a numeric interface, to test the machine. In this case to make sure the intensity of the radiation beams were uniform.

Considering the attention we were getting I found it difficult to understand what happened to a friend of mine a few years ago. When they discovered that he had prostate cancer he told me he was personally treated shoddily. He was not given any choice of treatment but simply told to report to the hospital for a radical prostatectomy. He said he was asleep for twelve hours after the procedure and when he woke up and asked how it went he was told, "tickety-boo." I could not find that medical term in any of the usual resources. As a result, he has been wearing what I believe is called a colostomy pouch, for the past few years. To make matters worse, his PSA is rising again and they want to do follow-up radiation therapy. He obviously feels he was severely damaged the first time and is reticent about going back to the same people for further treatment. I did my best to encourage him to agree to the treatment. Either the world has changed dramatically in a few years, or I am one lucky patient.

We left the meeting feeling pretty good and even though I was on my bland diet, I took Maureen to a sandwich shop and treated her to lunch.

8

One day my brother called me from Saint John, New Brunswick and said he found an interesting article on the *Globe and Mail* website. He read a quote to me over the phone: "A unique gene that can stop cancerous cells from multiplying into tumours has been discovered by a team of scientists at the B.C. Cancer Agency in Vancouver." I told him that it usually takes years before any practical applications become realistic. But there was one comment in the article that gave me some concern. It would appear that "if the gene in question is inactive then, when additional stress, such as radiation, is added, tumour growth is rampant."

This raised an interesting thought. Although there are many misconceptions about radioactivity it remains true that it is a carcinogen. It is not certain how dangerous it is to be treated with radiation, but it is thought that the cancer already in the body is far more threatening than the future effects of the radiation therapy.

The answer then seems to rest in the dose itself. If you sit in a tropical sun for one hour without protection you will probably get bad sunburn. But if you sit in the same sun for only 2 minutes a day for thirty days, you probably will not get sunburned. The difference is, the slow exposure gives the body a chance to heal any potential damage. The theory is that the normal cells that are damaged have the ability to repair themselves somewhat between treatments. So it may be true that large doses of radiation may cause cancer, but smaller doses are much less risky. Hence, that is why I receive it only five days a week and only 1.8 Gy per day. While this may be true not everyone agrees that is why the weekends are free of treatment. The real reason suggested is that it is a better approach to the workweek.

At this time I had completed twenty-seven treatments and I was nearing the beginning of a new program of radiation for the remaining fifteen days. This put my finishing date around the second week in September. Those remaining treatments concentrated on the prostate gland itself.

On one particular day I went into the room to change for treatment. Outside the Radiation area there are two change rooms, a toilet and a very small waiting room. The changing rooms have a bench at one end, a couple of hooks to hang clothes and a mirror to brush your hair and check the fall of your gown before heading off to see Linny.

When I came out of the change room that day, carrying my pants and underwear in the plastic bag, I intended to go and sit in the small waiting room. However, a dietitian, was consulting with two clients in the small treatment room, so I decided to hangout in the adjacent hall. She was the intern substitute because the earlier dietitian was away on vacation. I stood in the hall clutching my plastic bag and attempting to keep my gown modest as hospital staff rushed by. Soon after she came into the hall. When she finished speaking to her clients, I spoke to her. Immediately, she showed an interest, recalled my name, and asked how I was doing. She then invited me into the waiting room and asked me to describe my current diet. She wrote everything down on a sheet in her file and then asked if I was losing weight? I said I did not know. We arranged to meet after the radiation treatment. As soon as I was dressed she took me to a room near-by and recorded my weight. Again, I was amazed by the personal attention this hospital was providing me. She had come back down from her office in time to meet me after the radiation session. They know how to build confidence in those receiving treatment.

Fortunately, I had not lost any weight and she seemed satisfied. She also informed me that she was completing her internship and would be graduating the next day. I shook her hand and congratulated her as she left to return to her office on the fifteenth floor.

9

Finally another weekend and as usual we went to the boat. There happened to be a club race that day, and, even though exhausted I could not turn down an invitation to skipper a friend's vessel. I told him I was not able to grind winches or trim sails, but I could sit at the wheel and steer the boat. I did, and we did not do well in the race. However, he still speaks to me.

The next week got off to a slow start. Unit #4 was running thirty minutes late and this always created a problem with the bladder. I tried to get to the hospital each day about thirty minutes early, drink my water, and by the time they come to get me my bladder was full and I was ready for the shooting range. However, if the treatment time was delayed that meant I would have to either empty the bladder and wait even longer, or just hold on and hope for the best. Getting the timing on this exercise was very difficult and it took me most of the treatment period to figure it out. When there was an appointment delay, it compounded the problem and made it difficult to hold on to the bladder till the end of the treatment.

Also, at this time I was experiencing some diarrhea and this compounded the timing prior to treatment as well. I stopped taking the Milk of Magnesia as originally instructed, as I was not in need of any help. On the other hand if I took an Imodium, after a bout of diarrhea, I was unable to empty my bowels on time. So, on occasion, I would end up with a full bladder and full bowels. This was a constant problem. I found the best thing to do was to tell the radiation technologists whether I was ready or not.

Trying to find a solution to my plumbing difficulties resembled the arguments I had with myself at night. I was still getting up at least four times a night to tinkle. Originally when I woke up I stayed under the covers and argued with myself. If I could just hold on, I would think, perhaps I would go back to sleep and the urgency would pass. So I would lie there debating the pros and cons of the situation. Of course I would finally lose the argument, get out of bed, and go to the bathroom. Now that it had become a nightly occurrence, the senseless arguments gradually gave way to immediate action. I realized no matter how I argued with myself, the pressure to pee would always win. So, as soon as I woke up I climbed out of bed and trotted to the bathroom. It then took a long time to get back to sleep, but when I woke up the next time, no mental arguments, I just got on with the task. It was no wonder I was tired and felt at times like the mother of a newborn babe. I just wanted to get the routine finished, and back to some normalcy in my life. A booklet published by the Canadian Cancer Society recommends that you get up when you can't sleep and go to another room, read or watch TV until you start falling asleep, and then return to bed. However, I have a small portable radio with earplugs on the bed table. I plug in the earphones and listen to the CBC overseas programs. I usually fall asleep and wake up to the sound of the radio still plugged into my ears.

I was trying to relax on the boat on Sunday and suddenly I developed a severe case of diarrhea. A small boat with a tiny head (toilet) is not the place to hold a diarrhea session, so we packed up and headed home. That was the first real long session since the treatment began, and I was also experiencing severe pain each time I had to go to the bathroom. I tried the Sitz bath and changed into some comfortable clothes and, after a light dinner retired early.

After the Monday session that week, and the beginning of the new treatment, I had my weekly appointment with the doctor. We were having some outside doors replaced in our condominium and Maureen was not able to accompany me to the hospital. Once again the intern came into the treatment room where the consultations were usually held. I wanted to hear her understanding on radiation as a carcinogen. I suggested they were zapping the nasty cancer cells but were also creating a whole bunch of new devils in the process. She did not want to take time talking about possibilities and seemed only interested in the status of the side effects, the bowel and bladder functions. So she brushed off my general questions and then suggested a few remedies that I already knew. This occasion reinforced my realization how fortunate I was to have so many other staff that showed evidence they cared about the whole patient. I hoped that I was not judging her prematurely because she was an intern. After she left, the nurse came in and gave me my second shot of Lupron Depot. Lucky me, I can now look forward to more hot flashes, chills and night sweats.

On Tuesday when I was called to the treatment area the technologist gave me the weekly clipboard containing questions checking up on my plumbing system. They were certainly making every effort to see I was being looked after and to control any problems arising. I circled the severe diarrhea notation and let it go at that. On the way into the radiation room she wanted to talk about the problem and provided me with some excellent suggestions. I decided that, for some reason, the intern found it difficult to communicate with me, especially when Maureen was not present.

10

About this time I received an email from a friend who lives in British Columbia. He pointed out that since we were of similar vintage I should not be surprised that he recently learned that his PSA and Gleason scores were high. His GP recommended he see a specialist. He said the specialist only provided him with a textbook recitation and my friend wrote: "Even a travel agent gives you a possible itinerary but I found it remarkable that aside from some paper information I was given a report one might expect from a car mechanic." He was also led to believe, on his first visit, that he would become 'a sexless creature much like a eunuch'. What ever happened to the dictum: *Premium non-nocere* – First do no harm. No doubt he was afraid he would never be able to get his mojo working again. He was obviously not happy with what was going on, so I immediately emailed him back and gave him my best medical advice. In my opinion my comments surpassed the kind of information he was being fed which, in the end, was forcing him to think he was better off doing nothing. When he finally did see a written health report, he discovered that the doctor referred to him 'as a pleasant old fellow'.

We unreasonably expect our doctors to be prepared to answer all our questions. This expectation must be a strain, especially on young doctors, given the depth and breath of medical knowledge today. On the other hand, it is important for doctors to recognize the whole person, and not just our biological nature. I usually refer to myself, when making a call to a doctor's office, as a customer rather than a patient. As more and more people attempt to take charge of their health, mutual respect is paramount. 'Father doesn't always know best'. In England, doctors have to give clients a choice of four different hospitals they can approach for treatment. The client, or patient, is able to review how each hospital is performing in a number of critical areas. Is the hospital clean? What is its rate of acquired hospital infections? What will it cost? How long is the waiting time? And finally, is parking available? They probably should add: Are the doctors and staff, people or mechanics? This way the hospitals have to treat and respect their patients as customers. If they lose consumers, they lose funding.

My sister, a long retired hospital infection nurse, once told me with some alacrity, that if I got sick to stay out of the hospital. Today, some attention is now being given to her position on just how dangerous these institutions can be.

Hospital infections have been getting a lot of press in the past few years. A *CBC News Report* in 2005 said that super bug infections were spiraling out of control in Canadian hospitals. The two killers are Clostridium difficile (C. difficile) and methicillin-resistant staphylococcus aurus (MRSA). Another article even suggested bugs might kill as many as 8,000 patients a year in Canada and cost health-care systems at least $100 million annually. Joseph Brant Memorial Hospital in Burlington, Ontario recently admitted it lost 62 patients to C. difficile in a twenty month period. Unfortunately, Ontario and Quebec have the highest rates of C. difficile but recently things have been slightly improving in those provinces. Perhaps this is a problem for patients admitted to the hospital and not a concern for patients receiving day treatments. On the other hand, C. difficile travels from person to person through hand contact. That's why Maureen and I made sure we squirted on the sanitizer near the hospital entrance, both coming and going. One spokesperson even suggested we should ask any doctor examining us if they had washed their hands first. I was happy to read later that Princess Margaret Hospital was about to spend millions to control this situation, save lives and cut costs in the long run.

On Tuesday September 11, 2007, an infamous remembrance day in the United States, the *Globe and Mail* reported that the federal government would begin a national effort to reduce the scourge that is colonizing our hospitals. It pointed out that, up to the present day, the problem has been left to the individual hospitals. Dr. Donald Low, Microbiologist-in-Chief, Mount Sinai Hospital on a *CBC* morning newscast (October 18, 2007) said a recent U.S. study indicated the need for a new strategy in the United States. He said that study was also a wake-up call for Canadians. Obviously hygiene was listed as one of the most important solutions. Considering the harm being done, the washing of hands becomes a very important function for all hospital personnel. Sometimes, just doing simple things make big progress. It reminded me of a sign someone put near the hospital door: "Cancer Kills Smoking."

11

I get off the Don Valley South every day at Bloor Street and make a left turn onto Parliament Street. Then going west on Carleton St., I pass through what is known as 'The Discovery District' of Toronto. The Discovery District covers about a two and a half square kilometre area and is integrated into the downtown core. Located here is Canada's largest university, about twenty-four affiliated research institutes, and six research hospitals as well as 5,000 top scientists. The place is a brain magnet and many Canadian professionals have been lured back to the land of their birth. Most of the discoveries are in the bio-medical industry and there are over 700 companies involved in this industry. The mix includes bio-medical companies, finance and business support services. More than $500 million has currently been invested in the Medical and Related Sciences (MaRS) Centre. Princess Margaret Hospital is situated in the middle of this district.

Carleton Street, as it passes through this area, has bicycle paths on each side of the road. In the early morning there was always a stream of helmeted cyclists, wearing backpacks, moving east and west on their way to work. Dealing with the cabs, of which there seems to be hundreds, the general traffic and the bikes, makes it an interesting ride in the morning.

I hate to be late for an appointment and maneuvering through this morning conglomeration simply added to the stress of my journey. Even the streetcars and their slippery steel tracks provided an interesting challenge.

They stop at every intersection and open their doors for passengers. When the doors open, the vehicle drivers have to stop and unfortunately, this always seemed to happen when the light was green. When the light turned the drivers rushed to get in front of the streetcar before the next stop. Parked cars and construction vehicles parked along the side make the dash even more challenging. However, when you manage to get ahead of one streetcar, another seems to appear in the traffic ahead. This made it difficult for me at McCaul Street, where I had to make a left turn through the hordes of pedestrians who don't have the patience to wait for the proper light change.

The traffic was least when I had an early morning appointment. For example, if the appointment was at 8:00 AM I would leave the house at 6:30 AM. It usually took an hour to get to the hospital, so that gave me an opportunity to drink my water and then patiently wait until treatment time. However, when the appointments were later, I had to allow more time for rush hour stops and starts, along the way.

By now, on my unintended journey, I lost all claim to modesty. On one occasion when they were adjusting me on the Linear Accelerator bed, I pushed up with my arms, and again slipped on the paper covering. As I came down hard on the solid bed I felt my penis flip up from its usual place snugly tucked between my legs. It settled just shy of the tattoo spot over my prostate, the same spot they needed to see in order to adjust the bed. I did not attempt to move it back in place but simply waited to see how they would deal with the situation. One of the ladies simply folded the edge of the white sheet of paper quickly, made a little ridge near the fold, and quietly flipped my penis out of the way. No one said a word, but I found it difficult not to start laughing.

The radiation technologists changed frequently and it was difficult to keep the names straight. But one day one of the young ladies who sang to me on my birthday, came to get me in the waiting room. She quickly informed me that it was her birthday. I began to sing the Birthday Song for her as we walked along the hall. I was unable to complete the song when we entered the radiation room, as I had to identify myself and climb up on Linny. When the treatment was complete, I asked someone to tell me her age, as she was very young looking. I realized, however, that taking into consideration her education and training, I surmised that her looks might be deceiving. They asked me to guess.

She was 27 and I guessed 28. She said in a distressing voice: "Do I look 28 years old?" At that moment I think I lost a friend. I quickly said I took into consideration, not just her youthful looks, but her maturity and education. I am not sure that was a sufficient answer for me to save face.

On my way to the hospital every day I had to pass near the Bloor Street Bridge, but on the way home I had to pass over it. After the interstate bridge over the Mississippi River catastrophe earlier in the summer, I had a few misgivings about this daily trip over 490 metres of cement and steel suspended 40 metres above the valley below. Actually the valley the bridge crosses was, at one time, the ancient Lake Iroquois. The bridge is beautiful even with its Luminous Veil, a suicide barrier, to stop jumpers hurtling down on the Don Valley below.

There was even the theory that pigeons were responsible for the downfall of the Mississippi River Bridge. Decades of pigeon dung, or guano, had dried out to a salt and ammonia composite, which when mixed with water, promoted rust. I don't know any pigeons that roost below the Bloor Street Bridge, but I hope my few friends from the parking garage near the hospital, don't visit any relatives there. The span was completed in 1919 and no doubt many pigeons defecated and made love on its girders since then.

12

In spite of the Flomax and Lupron Depot, I was still getting up at least four times a night to visit the bathroom. On almost every occasion the awakening was prompted by a dream associated with the need to relieve my bladder. It was as if my brain was a movie screen onto which the camera was projecting colorful images. Of course, I was always in the lead role, fleeing danger or extreme discomfort. Those dreams were more vivid than I had ever experienced, and they deeply involved my emotions and senses. I don't remember this happening in the past, but it became a nightly intrusion while I was undergoing treatment. There is no doubt that the dreams were prompted by my physical need to pee. I think it was Freud who said dreams were a manifestation of our repressed longings and, his buddy Jung said they were a repressed wish. They got that right, but my repressed wish was simply to void my bladder. If nothing else, Freud and my dreams were about the same part of the human body. However, with due respect, Freud also once said: "Sometimes, a cigar is just a cigar." I felt my dreams were a sort of post-traumatic stress urging me to get up and go.

In one dream I was in an open, large dormitory, reminiscent of my early days in a boarding school. In my dream I got out of bed and wandered the halls surrounding the dorm, looking for a toilet. But in each washroom I entered, the restroom was either locked or disgustingly filthy and unusable. I went from floor to floor looking for one that I could use. I became frustrated and restless, and was at the point of despair of finding relief, when I would awaken with a start.

On another occasion I was sitting on the side of a hill. There were many other people picnicking on the sunny slope. As I wandered among them I realized I had to go to the bathroom, but I could not find anywhere private. Finally, I ask two female sunbathers to move the blanket they were sitting on. They stood up, and lifted their blanket off the grass. There, set in the ground, was a circular metal seat with a small hole in the middle. The girls were standing nearby, clutching their blanket and wondering what I was going to do. The other sunbathers became quiet and were staring at me. I just stood there and gazed at this strange toilet in the ground. I was too embarrassed to make use of the device and in desperation I woke up.

In one dream I was crawling through snow at the top of a bush-covered hill in desperate need of relief. Just as I was about to go crashing down the rock-strewn slope, I woke-up, saved by my bladder.

Then there was the time I dreamed that I was in uniform and part of a ceremony on a parade ground. Somehow or other the marching formation changed into a conga line and, as it circled around, I became more and more intertwined and confused, not knowing where I was supposed to go. I woke up and knew exactly where I had to go.

In almost every incident there is some sort of crisis prior to my waking up. It was never simply the raw urge to urinate, but always some related emergency that got me out of bed before calamity struck. I am still waiting for the dream about running water. But then again, that one may be too late.

On occasion the reality was worse than any of these strange dreams. For about a week, especially after they changed the radiation program, I had been feeling much better and even rested. In fact, I told the therapists one day that I had no need for Milk of Magnesia or Imodium tablets. I was still keeping faithfully to my diet and things were looking up.

After I reported this progress, I returned to the change room, left the hospital and got into my car and headed home. The trip was uneventful and I parked in my usual place in the underground. I boarded the elevator and pushed the button for the twentieth floor. No one else got on the elevator and that meant no stops on the way up. At around the tenth floor I began to feel an urge to go to the bathroom. I figured I would soon arrive at the apartment and tried to think of something else as I watched the floor numbers approaching twenty. All of a sudden my stomach roared and the urge to void my bowels became extremely urgent. I applied all of my will power and squeezed every muscle in my body to restrain myself. But to no avail. My damaged body was unable to control my need to defecate. Like the bursting of a volcano I pooped my pants. What a relief that no one else was on the elevator. I reached under my crotch with both hands to hold back the avalanche. The door of the elevator opened slowly and I crept down the hall toward our apartment door, clutching my pants with one hand, and reaching for my key with the other. My Mother used to say: "Did you have your movement today?" Yes, Mom, I had my movement today. She also told us to change our underwear daily 'in case you have to go the hospital'. How come mothers know so much?

I suppose the last time I did something like that was when I was a baby. What an embarrassment, especially after everything seemed to be going so well. It took me an hour to clean up and get my clothes into the washer. I am sure it gave a whole new meaning to Fruit of the Loom. After a warm shower and an Imodium pill I lay down on the couch thinking that there had been a sudden change in my progress. It was not only the discomfort I experienced, but also the new knowledge that things can change very quickly. That thought occupied my mind for the rest of the day.

The next day, on my way downtown, I got caught up in the early morning traffic. I was afraid there might be another occurrence with my bowels. I thought I should have thrown a spare pair of pants and underwear in the back of the car. But then, where would I clean up and change? If I had to pull over to the side of the highway I certainly would have become the reason for one great slowdown on the Don Valley Parkway, and an interesting moment on You Tube as half of Toronto stopped to see my bare bum. These imaginings were far worse than the nightly dreams. Thank God I made it safely to the hospital. I quickly crossed the foyer and entered the men's room. One of the two stalls was unoccupied, so I sat on the toilet and massaged my lower abdomen in an attempt to get some action before going down to the radiation waiting room. Fortunately, I had some success and felt better as I prepared for the treatment.

One of the technologists handed me the usual questionnaire and I marked that I had experienced that extraordinary event. We discussed it and decided to stick with the Imodium. I was told that if I wanted, they would put me in touch with the doctor after the treatment. I declined and said I would stick to the Imodium for the time being. I did ask them if other patients had to suffer the same mishap. They assured me they had and that I was not the first to face this embarrassment. Poor buggers.

On the way home I stopped at the gym for my exercise program. As I changed into my gym clothes I found myself talking to my underwear shorts. "I'm sorry for what happened yesterday and I will try not to let that happen again." I wonder if the other poor buggers ended up talking to their shorts as well. If they did, I bet they told no one about it.

13

There is one thing about these daily drives to downtown Toronto from Scarborough; I was learning a few things about the city. For example after I come off the Don Valley Parkway and turned down Parliament Street on my way to Cabbagetown, I drove through an area known as St. James Town. In the late 1800's it was an upper class area of the city with old Victorian homes. However in the 1950's almost all of the homes were torn down to make way for Toronto's first high-rise apartment towers, all eighteen of them. The apartments were intended for upwardly mobile singles, but in the end were populated by low or moderate-income families.

On the other side of this tree-lined street is St. James Cemetery, the oldest operating cemetery in Toronto. In the mid 1800's it was considered out in the countryside. Through the trees I could catch a glimpse of the beautiful St. James Chapel, which is known for its graceful spire. One day, as I drove down the street, the cemetery side was lined with huge white trucks belonging to a movie studio. I presume they were filming a scene in the graveyard. I wondered how many men, who are buried there, died of prostate cancer? They did not have the technology I was benefitting from and I hoped it would keep me out of there for some time to come. On the other hand, twenty years from now what will the technology be like, and how much simpler will it be to detect the problem and solve it quickly by tinkering with the genes? Perhaps someone will drive by my gravesite and think the same thoughts, how lucky they are to be still alive. Of course, they will only be lucky if their lives are qualitative and truly worth living. I know my life certainly has been.

When I am perched on Linny and everything is ready, the large modesty paper is placed discretely over my genitals, and the technologists then leave the room to start the treatment. There is usually a light breeze caused by the air conditioning. There was no breeze this particular day and they had no sooner started the procedure than some one turned on the air conditioner. I could feel my modesty paper begin to flutter. First, there was just a ripple effect and I never thought it might leave me bare, topside on the table. But it did, and the paper motions caused by the air stream increased. Suddenly, the paper took off and floated down to the floor. I started to giggle but did not move as I was told so many times. I knew there was nothing I could do about it so I waited, trying to control my own laughter, and wondered how it looked on the monitor in the control room. Then the machine stopped moving and making its usual noises, the door opened, and in came one of the technologists. She said: "That was the first time that happened. I think someone turned up the air conditioner." She threw an extra gown over me but could not contain her own giggles as she exited the radiation room. The door closed, and the procedure began once again. I had come a long way. Instead of being embarrassed, I just thought it was funny and remarked that the cool breeze felt good. As I was leaving to change back into my street clothes I said to the ladies in the control room, who were still in good spirits at their desks: "I hope I will not be arrested for flashing." I could still hear them laughing as I exited through the hallway ten minutes later.

At the very beginning of this journey I was concerned about modesty. After all, the cancer is in a traditionally protected area of my body that normally, as custom dictates, remains covered. As someone once wrote, why don't they find another place for the prostate? I avoid the word dignity as it brings up the notion of a moral concept or a legal term. The idea that a rational being, says E. Kant, has an intrinsic and absolute value, is not what I am concerned about here. The word dignity has a very broad application while modesty is individual and personal. There are organizations that deal with dignity such as *Dignity Canada/ Dignité* and *Dying with Dignity*. Nor is dignity a topic for discussion in Bioethics and the morality of medical treatments or actions that might help or harm by causing fear or pain. No, my sense of modesty probably stems from either my cultural or religious background. At any rate the only times that I had been previously publicly naked was during my annual checkup, or taking a shower after a session at the rink or gym. On those occasions I had not thought of modesty, shame or prudishness, I was just doing what had to be done. There was not fear of attracting undue attention to myself, especially my most intimate parts, which western culture says must be covered at all times in public.

In the beginning, all these visits with strangers and allowing them to examine me, or asking me to wear some strange garb was a source of some tension. After some forty days of treatment, being covered by the young ladies in the radiation room, and allowing them to adjust my body on the treatment bed, concern for modesty just did not cut it any longer, and I felt no embarrassment when the paper flew. I was able to experience the comical side of the event and join in the laughter with the others.

When I got home from the gym that day I checked my schedule for the next ten days and discovered there were only four days left for the treatment. I knew of at least one person who told me he quit before the treatments were complete. I figured the odds were in my favor and I was going to make it to the end. This knowledge gave me a little lift after what had happened the day before.

We had another summer long weekend, the Labour Day Weekend. Labour Day, a statutory holiday in Canada since the 1880's, always falls on the first Monday of September. Its origin goes back to the efforts of the eight-hour day movement, namely eight hours of work, eight hours of recreation, and eight hours of sleep. In the words of *All in the Family:* 'Those were the days my friends'. For us, as with most Canadians, it was the last long weekend of summer and a chance to spend some more time on the boat. I managed to get out for a few short sails, but by Monday I was so exhausted I simply sat in the shade on the back of the boat and read or dozed until it was time to return home.

14

The week following Labour Day was the beginning of the end of my treatments. After the usual session on Tuesday, Maureen and I visited with my oncologist. His assistant, was not around and although he was very busy, he was willing to deal with all of our concerns.

Obviously, this late in the sessions my first question had to be: What next? In a sense I had now come full circle. Did forty-two days of radiation catch the growth of cancer in my body? When was I going to find out if it worked?

Often prostate cancer starts in the gland cells and grows very slowly. It is difficult to say how slow or how fast it will develop. The doctor said it is not easy to detect the lumps because they are microscopic cancer cells. It appeared that I would have to wait three months before I would get another PSA test, and only then would they be able to get some idea of success. So we arranged to meet him again in early December of 2007. At that time I was also to get my third injection of Lupron Depot.

Our next question had to do with diet. No one told me I had to totally abstain from liquor, beer or wine. However, I thought it would be a good idea. I usually have some beer on the boat. Cold beer and sailing (only in port obviously) seem to go together. Early on in the treatments I decided a beer or two would not hurt on the weekend. However, I soon learned that beer only increased the number of times I had to get up at night, so it was not worth the trouble of pulling the tab. But the diet in general was very bland and I wanted to know how long after the treatment I would have to remain faithful to it?

I was telling a friend one day about the diet and pointed out that Maureen has lost six pounds on my diet. He thought that was very funny. Unfortunately, I did not lose weight, as the hormone treatment tends to add weight. So with the diet taking it off, and the hormones putting it on, I was staying within the same weight range. The doctor suggested that I stay on the diet for a couple of weeks, and then slowly work back to normal eating. He also said I could start taking my vitamins again in two weeks time. I knew the cause of fatigue was a combination of radiation, hormones and the nightly crawls to the bathroom, but I always felt better when I added a few vitamins to my daily intake. So whatever fatigue was a result of the radiation will obviously diminish after the treatments stop. The fatigue caused by the hormone treatment will continue for about three years. He also said I should continue with the calcium and vitamin D.

The next question we posed had to do with the nature of the damage done by the radiation. Would there be any permanent damage, scar tissue for example, to healthy organs? He divided the question into acute side effects and chronic side effects. I figured the word acute means sudden, but of a short term. In other words, there was some damage, but we would have to wait approximately five or six months to see if the acute side effects become chronic. Chronic means of long duration or even permanent. So I would have two more things to worry about: First, were they able to kill off all those little cancer buggers? And second: will the damage to my bowel and bladder ever come to an end? I guess I was back to the discussion on doing no harm.

The Clinical Research Study I joined was to compare the standard therapy with the treatment I had been receiving. My doctor said there were 58 men left of the 60 who started the current study. He also wanted to find out if receiving a higher dose of radiation to the prostate and lymph nodes and, the same or a milder dose of radiation to the normal body tissues, would reduce the possible side effects. So he was a little concerned that I did have a few bad episodes, especially with my bowels. He hoped to recruit another hundred and fifty volunteers and show that the side effects are indeed less than they are in conventional therapy. If he can show that, this program could become the norm in the future.

Finally, I asked him how much my treatment was costing. I had tried to do some research, but it is difficult to pin down any numbers as there are so many permutations and combinations of procedures, people, and machines. The Ontario government is spending more that $40 billion a year and there is no indication that the costs will slow down. He said that based on an American study it could be in the vicinity of $300,000. I don't think I am moving to the U. S. any time soon. Of course that number does not include parking, gas, time, inconvenience and embarrassment. I will never have a negative thing to say about the Canadian Health Care System again.

At the same time I finally figured out why old people get sick: we are the only ones who have the time to keep all the appointments and run around town for treatments.

15

At last the final day of treatment arrived. Unfortunately, for the first time, I had to change the appointment on the schedule. I was also seeing a dermatologist regarding sunspots. However, each time I cancel with him the next available appointment was six to ten weeks later. Some of the spots were getting nasty and I did not want to put this off until a later time. I explained that to the technologist and she happily adjusted my appointment time to late in the afternoon. It was unfortunate that the very last time slot had to be changed, but I figured I could not wait any longer.

I went to the dermatologist at 11:30 AM. I decided, because of the parking problems, to take my car to Fairview Mall and go downtown on the subway. The dermatologist's office was about half way down Yonge Street so I could get off there and, when he was done, take the tube the rest of the way down to the hospital.

Since I had a few hours to fill after seeing the dermatologist, I took the subway to the huge Eaton Centre and then went up to street level. There was a large crowd gathered in the Yonge-Dundas Square. This Square is a relatively new addition to downtown Toronto. A block of buildings was removed to make a gathering place. Large screens were projecting images so that the people in the square could follow the proceedings in the square below. Many events throughout the year take place here such as free concerts, Christmas specials and film screenings. There is a stage at one end and, on this particular day a number of performers were entertaining over a thousand people gathered in the square. Most were wearing red ball caps marked United Appeal. The social assistance organizations that benefit from the United Appeal were present in groups advertising their services with large signs and different colored T-shirts that sported the name of their organization.

I removed my ball cap, stuffed it in my knapsack and donned a red cap offered me as I approached the square. Around the edge of the square were small kiosks selling various types of sandwiches, pop, cookies and salads. I bought what I thought were oatmeal cookies only to find they also contained raisins. I ate them anyway.

From there I wandered over to the Eaton Centre to do some window-shopping. Eventually, I found my way to Nathan Phillips Square and Toronto's big clam City Hall. Nathan Phillips was the mayor of Toronto from 1955 to 1962. The square promotes many special events as well, such as the New Year Eve celebrations. There is a peace garden and a famous or infamous statue called the Archer by the British sculptor Henry Moore. A reflecting pool with arches, becomes a skating rink in the winter season. A speaker's corner has a statue of Winston Churchill nearby. One interesting aspect of this square at City Hall is the parking lot under it that has room for two thousand four hundred cars. When I first exited the Eaton Centre, on my way to the Nathan Phillips Square, I did not know where I was. I later learned the building near where I exited, was at the back of the old city hall.

This square was busy with a police graduation and up on the stage were the dignitaries including the mayor of Toronto. I watched the proceedings for about ten minutes; it was hot, and even though early in the day I decided to head for the hospital. There I knew I would find a cool place to settle down and read my book as I waited for final visit with Linny, the Linear Accelerator.

I was two hours early for my last treatment so I found a comfortable seat near the Japanese Garden and found a cool and quiet corner to read. About an hour later I wandered into the smaller waiting area and checked in on the computer only to learn Unit #4 was running thirty minutes late. I settled down with my book again but also watched the patients come and go. A volunteer came around with juice and cookies, so I had a second lunch. There were as many women in this waiting area as there were men that day. The surrounding hallway resembled a busy street. Patients in wheel chairs or gurneys were being moved into the radiation rooms. One man sitting nearby told his companion that they were hospital patients and they were jumping the day patients waiting line, thus the delay.

At one point I glanced up from my book and, to my surprise, saw Maureen coming down the busy corridor. She said she was concerned about the heat and my traveling on the subway and came to drive me back to Fairview Mall where my truck was parked. I convinced her that it was going to be a very long wait and finally she decided to head home and think about dinner. This was a good decision as she left around 2:30 PM but I did not get in for treatment until 3:45 PM.

The treatment went well and when it was over I handed the technologist a card with a note of appreciation I had written. I promised her that I would get the results of their work to them after December 11, 2007. I don't know if they ever find out if their dedicated work is successful or not. Do they just keep doing their job day after day without feedback? She seemed to appreciate the card, but I did not have an opportunity to speak to her later. Fortunately, I met one of the technologists in the hall on the way out and she told me she had been moved to another unit. We spoke for a few minutes and then I was on my way out of there.

16

The Unintended Journey was half over. I had reached my destination, but would I be a passenger on the return trip? Going to the hospital five days a week for the summer was indeed similar to having a job. Not only was I tired from the diet imposed on me, but also rest did not ameliorate radiation fatigue. I was looking forward to real meals, and even something as simple as taking my vitamins again as I waited for the results of the treatments.

My next appointment with the doctor was set for December 11, 2007. At that time he would report the results of the radiation and I would receive the third injection of Lupron Depot. A week prior to my visit I had to get another PSA test providing him with some conclusive results.

Unfortunately, I found myself back in never-never land, worried about results and, beginning another long period of waiting. I was hoping we had made some progress through all those long summer days.

I slowly returned to a more normal diet. On one or two occasions I overdid it and paid the consequences. That Scotch drink I was longing for finally happened, but I paid the price and was up half the night as a result. Friends started telling me I was looking better. Strange, they never told me I looked bad. I suppose they were trying to encourage and support my experience with cancer. At the same time I had to admit I was feeling better. After the prescribed two-week waiting period I started taking my multivitamins again. I began to experience a slow restoration of my energy level and upped my visits to the gym from two to three days a week.

I did not really know what to expect from this Unintended Journey. I was told that many men are cured. I still found it difficult to believe there is such a thing as a cure for cancer, any cancer. In my mind, and what I hoped for, was that the disease had been given a setback and would not push itself front and center for a few more years. In the meantime, I joined the watchful waiters and returned to my pre-journey life.

If nothing else, the journey helped me focus on the limitations of my own existence. I realized the end was definitely on the horizon, but at the same time it gave me a better understanding of that simple fact: all life ends at one point or another. There was nothing negative or depressing about this realization. It simply meant that from that day on I could focus more on making every day more special and exciting.

17

It was now necessary to wait a few months for the radiation to leave my body and to return for another consultation with the oncologist. The date was set for December 11, 2007, approximately three months later because the PSA could not be measured too soon after radiation. I found myself becoming more anxious as the day approached. I thought the days of Sitz baths and cranberry juice would end, but they did not. I ran out of Flomax, and my nightly visits, of approximately two or three a night, continued.

During this time I was anxious to know if the treatment worked as planned. In my own mind, as mentioned, I never expected a cure from cancer. What I hoped for was that the treatment would provide me with the ability to outlive the disease, that I would die *with* it, not *of* it. At the same time, I knew the hormone injections would play a major role in that hope. The continued hormone injections, with their negative side effects, are much more desirable than the alternative, dying of cancer.

One of the effects of the radiation was hair loss. I did not expect this nor did I find anything in the literature that indicated this would happen. However, the loss was not on my head. One day when lounging in the tub, enduring my Sitz bath, I thought I was putting on weight. Suddenly, I realized what was different was that my pubic hair had disappeared. How was I to explain that in the change room at the gym?

The problem of night visits to the bathroom remained unsolved. I renewed the prescription for Flomax. However, I still found it necessary to visit the bathroom every two and a half hours. Hence, I was unable to get a full night's sleep. I tried a little brandy before going to bed, but all it did was increase the number of visits. The discouraging aspect of these nightly itinerant travels was that quantitatively they did not amount to much. I felt each visit was a waste of time, and yet I had to make the trek if I wanted to fall back to sleep. This was a habit I could not break.

In early November Maureen and I decided to take a vacation and we booked a flight to St. Maarten and stayed at Guana Bay for two weeks. The first week we were joined by two of Maureen's sisters. The second week I spent the whole time sitting on a chair under an umbrella reading mystery stories, taking long walks on the beach, and spending hours in the warm Atlantic water. The only bad thing I did was getting too much sun and perhaps a little too much rum as well.

By the end of September, I no longer needed to take the cranberry juice to alleviate the burning sensation when urinating, nor was it necessary to take the Sitz bath. However, the second week in St. Maarten those aggravations slowly reared their ugly heads, and once again cranberry juice and Sitz baths were necessary. In the latter case I gave up using my plastic seat over the toilet bowel, and decided to bathe in the bathtub instead. Fortunately, I did not have to do this every day, but at least two or three times a week.

As we approached the December meeting I found myself more and more tense. Ennui was settling in. I found myself thinking, I have had a long and happy life, unlike so many other poor people in the world, and if I were to die soon, it would not be a great tragedy. These feelings usually were aroused in the early morning as I lay in bed summoning up the energy to start another day.

On the Tuesday one week prior to the appointment with the oncologist, I returned to the blood lab at the Princess Margaret Hospital in order to generate a PSA report for the following week.

Finally December 11, 2007 arrived. I was pulling into the station house and wondered: Would the doctor have a ticket waiting for me to return on my Unintended Journey?

18

On December 11, 2007, I woke up earlier than usual and tried listening to my MP3 player, with earplugs, in bed. However, I was restless and finally got up, made a pot of coffee, and retired to the living room with the *Globe and Mail*. The weather was not promising and I was not sure whether to take the subway to the hospital or to attempt to drive. Since our appointment was not until three-thirty in the afternoon, I figured the weather would be settled one way or the other before then. The forecast predicted rain, turning to freezing rain, and that does not make for good driving.

After breakfast I prepared some questions to ask the doctor. I made two columns; one if we discovered the treatment was not a success, and the other if it was successful. Of course, our first question was to get the results of the latest PSA blood test.

We left our underground parking space at 2:00 PM and when we were on the road we discovered that the light snow was not accumulating on the ground and the streets were wet, but not slippery with ice. Hence, we decided to drive to the hospital.

We parked the car in the church parking lot and walked over to the entrance to Princess Margaret Hospital. There were a few changes since September, more construction fences were built around the front and part of the street was fenced off. Other than that, nothing appeared to have changed as we entered the hospital foyer and proceeded up to the fourth floor and the Prostate Centre. We were a half hour early and I handed in my Health Card and Hospital Card to the clerk at the desk and we took a seat in the familiar, but very crowded waiting area. Our anxiety was building and I kept glancing toward the area where my doctor conducted his examinations. Three-thirty came and went and each time his assistant appeared at the front desk I thought she was there to call us. We learned later there had been some problem arranging appointments, and they had overbooked. Maureen watched the various patients and their companions coming and going. We started reading the magazines on the coffee table and discussing the food recipes in the Chatelaine magazines. I wondered why there were so many magazines geared to women on the table in the Prostate Centre?

The room gradually cleared out and finally we were called to the treatment room at about 5:00 PM. I handed her the Lupron Depot injection I had brought from the drugstore and we sat down to wait. The oncologist came in and in spite of the heavy workload that day he immediately produced a sheet with the PSA results. It showed the following: before treatment the PSA test on February 22, 2007 was 6.40, by April 19, 2007 it had increased to 6.62. However, the final result after all the treatments was less than 0.22. This was the result we were hoping for. He then pulled the curtain on the examination table and he proceeded with a short physical test that included the DRE. He announced that the prostate no longer had bumps but was smooth.

We took this to mean that the cancer was now under control and that the external radiation therapy was a success. We then proceeded to ask him the prepared questions and he certainly encouraged me to continue my exercise routine and indicated there was no problem getting out the skis again that winter.

After our discussion I thanked him and asked him to convey the final information to the radiation technologists. I had promised them that I would let them know the results of their hard work, but since it was too late that day to go down stairs, I asked him if he would pass on the good news. He promised to do that for us.

After he left, his assistant came into the room and administered the hormone injection. I noticed on the package containing the luteinizing hormone-releasing hormone (LHRH), that there were 10 treatments remaining. Since these treatments are given every four months I figured I had about three years of treatment left. Hormone treatment is not a local therapy but rather, a systemic treatment, it treats the whole body and not just a particular area. As mentioned before, it deprives

Dick Grannan

the prostate cancer cells of the androgens they need to survive. An alternative would be surgical removal of the testicles.

Hence, hormone therapy does not cure prostate cancer, and the side effects I have never become comfortable with, will continue: the sweating, hot flashes, night chills, no sex drive, loss of body hair and some minor mood swings. But think of the alternative?

It is possible that cancer can stop responding to hormone therapy and the PSA will start to rise again. However, given my age, it will probably work long enough so that when the time comes I will die of some other cause.

We left the hospital in good spirits and shortly after met a number of our friends and gave them the good news. It would appear, at least for now, that I have been given the ticket for my return trip. The Unintended Journey has been successful.

References

Baker, G. Ross et al. "Canadian Adverse Events Study: The incidence of adverse events among hospital patients in Canada." *Canadian Medical Association Journal*, May 25, 2004.

Bristow, Robert G. "DNA Repair and Genetic Instability in Solid Tumours." Feb. 5, 2007.
www.uhnres.utoronto.ca/researchers/profile.php?lookup=645.

"Canadian Team Discovers Gene That Turns Cancer Off." *Globe and Mail,* August 13, 2007.

College of Family Physicians of Canada. "The College of Family Physicians of Canada Takes Action to Improve Access to Care for Patients in Canada." *News Release,* October 11, 2007.

Davis, Devra. *The Secret History of the War on Cancer.* New York: Basic Books, 2007.

Foxman, Stuart. "Maintaining Boundaries." College of Physicians and Surgeons of Ontario, *Dialogue,* September 6, 2007.

Fraser, John. "The Way We Mourn." *Maclean's,* September 3, 2007.

Groopman, Jerome. *How Doctors Think.* Boston-New York: Houghton Mifflin, 2007.

Johnson, Carla. CT Scans Don't Cut Smokers' Deaths from Lung Cancer." *Globe and Mail*, March 7, 2007.

"Making it Better: Curing Canada's Top Cancer Facility." *Toronto Star*, April 13, 2007.

"N.S. gets millions for wait-time guarantees." *Canadian Press*, March 26, 2007.

Picard, André. "More Men Need Prostate Cancer Testing." *Globe and Mail*, September 12, 2007.

Priest, Lisa. "Government Initiatives Target Super Bugs." *Globe and Mail*, September 11, 2007.

"Superbug's Infections Spiraling in Canadian Hospitals." *CBC News*, March 23, 2005. www.cbc.canada/story/2005/03/21infection-canada050321.

"There's Nothing to These Waiting-time Guarantees." *Globe and Mail*, April 2, 2007.

U.S. Department of Health and Human Services. Agency for Healthcare Research and Quality. *Reducing Errors in Health Care: Translating Research Into Practice*. AHRQ Publication No. 00-PO58, April 2000.

"Waiting Times to Receive Care Under Canada's National Health System in 2006." *Lebanon Daily News*, March 26, 2007.

SUGGESTED READING:

1. Jones, J. Stephen. *The Complete Prostate Book:: What every Man Needs to Know: Benign Problem, Prostate Enlargement, Reducing Your Risk of Cancer, Sexual Health, Latest Treatments for Prostate Cancer*. Amherst, N.Y.: Prometheus Books, 2005.

2. Trachtenberg, John, Neil Fleshman, Carol Lancaster and Barbie Casselman. *Eating Right for Life. Prostate Cancer Nutrition & You*. Montreal: Parkhurst, 2000. (Available at Patient and Family Library, Princess Margaret Hospital, Toronto.)